The Which? Guide to Complementary Therapies

About the author

Helen Barnett is a member of Consumers' Association's *Drug and Therapeutics Bulletin* team. A pharmacist by training, she is also a lay representative on the Committee on Safety of Medicines (CSM). In addition, she is a practising acupuncturist and has an MSc in Complementary Therapy Studies, which included studying the integration of complementary and conventional medicine.

Acknowledgements

The author and publisher would like to thank Professor Edzard Ernst (University of Exeter) and Professor Adrian Furnham (University College, London) for their valuable advice and helpful comments on the manuscript.

We are indebted to the following individuals or organisations for their comments.

Acupuncture: British Acupuncture Council, British Medical Acupuncture Society, Acupuncture Association of Chartered Physiotherapists. **Alexander technique**: Society of the Teachers of Alexander Technique. **Aromatherapy**: Aromatherapy Trade Council. **Autogenic therapy**: British Autogenic Society. **Biofeedback**: Biofeedback Foundation of Europe. **Chiropractic**: General Chiropractic Council, McTimoney Chiropractic Association. **Healing**: Confederation of Healing Organisations. **Herbal medicine**: Ayurvedic Medical Association, British Ayurvedic Medical Council. **Homeopathy**: Faculty of Homeopathy and British Homeopathic Association, Society of Homeopaths. **Hypnotherapy**: British Society of Medical and Dental Hypnosis, National Register of Hypnotherapists and Psychotherapists. **Massage therapy**: London School of Sports Massage, Shiatsu Society. **Naturopathy**: British Naturopathic Association. **Nutritional therapy**: Sue Davies and Nikki Ratcliff (Consumers' Association). **Osteopathy**: General Osteopathic Council, Craniosacral Therapy Association of UK. **Reflexology**: Association of Reflexologists, International Federation of Reflexologists, Reflexology Forum, Reflexologists' Society. **Relaxation therapy and meditation techniques**: Friends of the Western Buddhist Order, School of Meditation, Transcendental Meditation. **Yoga**: Veronica Gould (British Wheel of Yoga), Roz Peters (Yoga Therapy Centre), Iyengar Yoga Institute.

Dowsing: British Society of Dowsers. **Kinesiology**: Kinesiology Federation. **Art therapy**: British Association of Art Therapists. **Bowen technique**: Bowen Therapists European Register. **Chelation therapy**: Arterial Health Foundation. **Crystal healing**: Affiliation of Crystal Healing Organisations. **Dance and drama therapy**: Association for Dance Movement Therapy. **Feldenkrais method**: Feldenkrais Guild UK. **Flower remedies**: Dr Edward Bach Centre. **Hellerwork**: European Hellerwork Association. **Holotropic breathwork**: British Rebirth Society. **Magnetic therapy**: British Biomagnetic Association. **Metamorphic technique**: Metamorphic Association. **Music therapy**: British Society for Music Therapy. **Rolfing**: Rolf Institute. **T'ai chi and Qigong**: T'ai Chi Union. **Tragerwork**: Trager UK.

The Which? Guide to Complementary Therapies

Helen Barnett

 CONSUMERS' ASSOCIATION

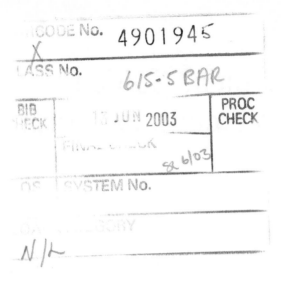
Which? Books are commissioned and researched by
Consumers' Association and published by
Which? Ltd, 2 Marylebone Road, London NW1 4DF
Email address: books@which.net

Distributed by The Penguin Group:
Penguin Books Ltd, 80 Strand, London WC2R 0RL

First edition October 2002

Copyright © 2002 Which? Ltd

Based on *The Which? Guide to Complementary Medicine* by Barbara Rowlands.

British Library Cataloguing in Publication Data
A catalogue record for this book is available from the British Library

ISBN 0 85202 893 8

For a full list of Which? books, please write to Which? Books, Castlemead, Gascoyne Way,
Hertford X, SG14 1LH, or access our website at www.which.net

Editorial and production: Joanna Bregosz, Lynn Bressler, Nithya Rae
Cover photograph: David Gifford/Science Photo Library

Typeset by Saxon Graphics Ltd, Derby
Printed and bound in Great Britain by Creative Print and Design (Wales), Ebbw Vale

Contents

Part III   Diagnostic techniques and other therapies

★An asterisk next to the name of an organisation in the text indicates that the address or website can be found in this section

Foreword

Complementary therapies have become more and more important, mainly because consumers are embracing them with growing enthusiasm. Today it is almost politically incorrect to oppose aspects of complementary medicine.

This type of uncritical acceptance is in danger of causing harm in the long run. What the field needs, like any other branch of medicine, is a healthy dose of constructive criticism. Without it, complementary medicine will come and go as any other health fad before it. So critical analysts have to ask questions like 'Does it really work beyond a placebo response?', 'Is it safe?', 'Does it do more good than harm?' and 'How does it compare to conventional treatment options?'. Only through asking these probing questions can progress be made.

But these are uncomfortable questions for those – both consumers and providers – who believe in complementary medicine. And because they are awkward they are frequently brushed aside. *The Which? Guide to Complementary Therapies* stands out as one of the few consumer books that makes an honest attempt to provide the answers based on facts and current best knowledge.

Complementary medicine is much more consumer-driven than most other branches of medicine. Consumers should therefore make their voices heard in a constructive way: in particular they should insist that some public funds are channelled towards studies of complementary therapies. The future of complementary medicine critically depends on the intensity of research in years to come.

I am delighted to see *The Which? Guide to Complementary Therapies*, not least because it is refreshingly different from the plethora of promotional, uncritical texts. I am hopeful that, provided research intensifies, the next edition will be an even more informative book for the benefit of the consumer.

Professor Edzard Ernst
Department of Complementary Medicine, University of Exeter
Author of *The desktop guide to complementary and alternative medicine*

Introduction

Broadly speaking, complementary therapies are those healthcare practices not currently an integral part of conventional medicine. However, the approaches taken by the two types of medicine are overlapping more and more. Concepts historically associated with complementary therapies, such as holistic healthcare, the mind-body link, 'energy' or vitalism, and self-healing, are beginning to permeate conventional medicine. An exciting development is the notion of 'integrated healthcare', which combines complementary and conventional medicine and is gaining interest in many circles, from general practice to academia.

Complementary therapies are more popular in the UK today than ever before, with an estimated 4–5 million people seeing a therapist each year. And most people using such therapies generally seem to be satisfied with their treatment; when asked in a survey conducted by *Which?* in 2001, 64 per cent of 1,198 subscribers said they were very satisfied and only 3 per cent wanted to complain about a therapist. The reasons for the rise in popularity vary, and seem to be both negative (such as disillusionment with certain aspects of conventional medicine) and positive (the fact that so many people claim to have benefited from it). Moreover, research suggests that most people tend to use non-orthodox therapies *alongside* conventional medicine, rather than as an alternative to it.

There are increasing numbers of people practising complementary medicine. From 1981 to 1997, the number of non-medically qualified registered practitioners trebled to about 50,000. In addition, the number of medically qualified healthcare practitioners using complementary therapies has risen too.

The use of complementary medicine is also on the up worldwide, which is reflected in the first global 'Traditional Medicine Strategy' published by the World Health Organisation (WHO) for the period 2002-5. According to WHO, the global market for traditional therapies is currently around $60 billion per year, and is growing steadily.

This upsurge in popularity of complementary therapies has resulted in moves to regulate the field more closely, primarily to safeguard public health, and to increase research into their effectiveness. Recently, Acts of Parliament have established statutory self-regulation for chiropractic and osteopathy, with the acupuncture, herbal medicine and homeopathy professions likely to follow suit soon. The report on complementary and alternative medicine by the House of Lords Select Committee on Science and Technology, published in late 2000, concluded that better regulation of complementary therapies is essential to protect the needs of the public. In its response to the report, the government stated that complementary medicine has a role to play within the NHS but must meet the same standards as other NHS treatments.

Moves are also afoot at European level to regulate complementary medicine, such as the EU Directive on traditional herbal medicinal products, which will require all over-the-counter medicines made from herbal ingredients to be licensed, in order to ensure safety and quality.

The therapies in this book have been examined, as far as possible, with a critical eye. Many of them have little science to back them up, but appear to work none the less. Unlike books written on the subject by people with a vested interest in putting over a particular view, this guide takes an independent look at the therapies people are most likely to come into contact with. Most practitioners are well aware that they still have to prove to the world at large that their therapies work. They are beginning to do so now, with an ever-increasing body of scientific research to back up their claims. Such research is to be welcomed, as is the regulation of the industry, in order to protect public health and to arm consumers with the information they need to make informed choices about the best treatments for their circumstances.

Please note that although this book provides medical information, it is essential that you consult your GP for specific advice.

Chart of conditions and suitable therapies

This chart is not comprehensive but gives a guide to the complementary therapies that have been shown, in at least one well-conducted trial, to benefit the common conditions listed here. This does not necessarily mean that no other complementary therapies work for these conditions, nor that there are no effective complementary therapies for health problems not listed here. Generally, it simply indicates that no well-controlled trials have been conducted in these or other areas for other complementary therapies.

Acne	**Aromatherapy (tea tree oil)**
Addiction	**Acupuncture (except for smoking)**
Asthma	**Hypnotherapy** **Relaxation (breathing exercises)** **Yoga**
Back pain	**Acupuncture** **Alexander technique** **Chiropractic** **Herbal medicine (devil's claw)** **Massage** **Osteopathy** **Yoga**
Benign prostatic hyperplasia	**Herbal medicine (saw palmetto,** **African plum, nettle)**
Cancer (palliative care)	**Acupuncture** **Healing** **Hypnotherapy** **Massage/aromatherapy**
Congestive heart failure	**Herbal medicine (hawthorn)**

Constipation	Biofeedback Herbal medicine (senna) Massage
Depression (mild to moderate)	Herbal medicine (St John's wort) Relaxation therapy
Diabetes	Naturopathy Yoga
Eczema	Chinese herbal medicine Hypnotherapy
Erectile dysfunction	Herbal medicine (yohimbine)
Hay fever	Homeopathy
Headache	Biofeedback Chiropractic Hypnotherapy Osteopathy
Heart disease (reducing risk factors, e.g. high cholesterol levels)	Herbal medicine (hawthorn, garlic, guar gum) Naturopathy Nutritional therapy (oat fibre, psyllium)
High blood pressure	Biofeedback Naturopathy Relaxation and meditation Yoga
Incontinence	Biofeedback
Insomnia	Herbal medicine (valerian) Relaxation therapy
Irritable bowel syndrome	Hypnotherapy Herbal medicine (peppermint)
Memory loss/Alzheimer's	Herbal medicine (*Gingko biloba*)
Menopausal symptoms	Herbal medicine (black cohosh, chaste tree) Naturopathy/nutritional therapy (soya-rich foods) Relaxation therapy
Migraine	Acupuncture Herbal medicine (feverfew) Relaxation therapy
Nausea and vomiting	Acupuncture/acupressure Herbal medicine (ginger)
Neuralgia	Acupuncture

Osteoarthritis	Acupuncture Herbal medicine (devil's claw, willow bark) Supplements (glucosamine, chondroitin) Yoga
Peripheral arterial disease	Herbal medicine (*Gingko biloba*)
Pre-menstrual syndrome	Biofeedback Naturopathy Reflexology
Raynaud's phenomenon	Biofeedback
Ringworm/athlete's foot	Aromatherapy (tea tree oil)
Stress/anxiety	Biofeedback Hypnotherapy Meditation Relaxation therapy
Stroke	Acupuncture
Tennis elbow	Acupuncture
Urinary tract infections	Herbal medicine (echinacea, cranberries) Nutritional therapy (vitamin C)

It is a good idea to consult your doctor before trying a complementary therapy, particularly if you have a diagnosed disease, are taking any prescribed drugs, have any symptoms of illness, or if you are pregnant or are trying to conceive. Do not stop taking any prescribed drugs without first consulting your doctor, and always check with a pharmacist, doctor or registered herbalist first before taking a herbal remedy with any other medicine (prescribed or bought over the counter), as they may interact. If your symptoms persist or get worse while you are having a complementary therapy, consult your doctor.

Part I

Complementary therapies – an overview

Chapter 1

What are complementary therapies?

There is no one definition of what complementary therapies are, because the definition needs to encompass a diverse collection of ancient and modern beliefs. Broadly speaking, complementary therapies are those healthcare practices that are not currently an integral part of conventional medicine. However, which therapies are considered to be complementary or alternative is not fixed; new therapies are constantly being developed and, as a therapy is shown to be effective and safe, it can become accepted as a conventional healthcare practice (for example, as is happening with chiropractic and osteopathy). Commonly, now, the practice of complementary therapies is referred to as complementary and alternative medicine (CAM) or just complementary medicine. Here we use these terms synonymously. Other terms, which have now fallen out of favour, used to describe this collection of therapies include unorthodox, unconventional or fringe therapies. A new term is integrated healthcare (see page 30).

The Cochrane Collaboration (an organisation providing systematic reviews of controlled trails; see page 58) defines complementary and alternative medicine as: '… a broad domain of healing resource that encompasses all health systems, modalities, and practices and their accompanying theories and beliefs, other than those intrinsic to the politically dominant health system of a particular society or culture in a given historical period. CAM includes all such practices and ideas self-defined by their users as preventing or treating illness or promoting health and well-being. Boundaries within CAM and between the CAM domain and that of the dominant [conventional] system are not always sharp or fixed.'

It is difficult, if not impossible, to find defining criteria that are common to all complementary therapies. Several attempts at some sort of classification have been made. The main categories that have been suggested are the following:

1. Alternative medical systems (for example, Ayurveda, Traditional Chinese Medicine (TCM)). These include healthcare systems that have evolved in the context of a society's culture, and which are completely different from the conventional 'Western' system.

2. Complete systems of healing (for example, TCM acupuncture, chiropractic, herbal medicine, homeopathy, naturopathy, osteopathy). This category includes therapies that have a comprehensive theoretical background and are able to treat most presenting conditions within the system. Often, they will have their own explanation for causes of disease and mechanism for treating them.

3. Mind-body interventions (for example, hypnotherapy, meditation, yoga, visualisation). These are interventions that recognise the link between the mind and the body.

4. Biologically based treatments (for example, aromatherapy, herbal medicine, naturopathy). These include therapies that are aimed, although not necessarily exclusively, at changing the physiology of the body.

5. Manipulative and structural therapies (for example, chiropractic, osteopathy, rolfing, yoga).

6. Postural techniques (for example, Alexander technique, Feldenkrais method, yoga).

7. Touch-based therapies (for example, massage, shiatsu, metamorphic technique, reflexology, Tragerwork, aromatherapy).

8. Energy therapies (for example, Ayurveda, TCM acupuncture, reflexology, yoga). This includes therapies that are aimed at changing the 'energy' of the body.

9. Specific therapeutic methods (for example, healing, massage, reflexology). These are therapies that are techniques rather than whole systems of healing. It is possible to use treatment methods from the latter in this way, such as using acupuncture techniques outside the context of the system of TCM.

10. Diagnostic methods (for example, hair analysis, iridology).

11. Self-care approaches (for example, meditation, nutrition, yoga).

Many of the therapies can be placed in more than one category. Others have superficial similarities in philosophy but are, in fact, quite distinct; for example, reflexology and metamorphic technique are both concerned with the feet, but there the similarity ends. Acupuncture and yoga are both concerned with energy systems, but vary in the way that the energy is boosted. So, ideally, each therapy needs to be approached individually.

Therapies differ markedly in the techniques they employ and their approach to the human body. Some involve direct intervention by way of pills or potions (herbalism) or the manipulation of the body (chiropractic); others, such as healing, involve the laying-on of hands. A few, such as radionics, do not even require the patient's physical presence.

The aims of the therapies and the ways in which they are practised also vary. Some techniques, such as kinesiology and iridology, are seldom used as stand-alone therapies but as tools by practitioners of other therapies. Many therapies, such as Chinese herbal medicine, are mainly used to help treat specific conditions, while others, such as aromatherapy, are used mainly to promote a general sense of well-being. Therapies such as yoga and t'ai chi can be practised in groups or alone; others, such as osteopathy, involve being treated by the practitioner on a one-to-one basis.

Concepts associated with complementary therapies

There are certain concepts that are perceived as being characteristic to all complementary therapies, and which are often thought not to apply to conventional medicine. Although the approaches of conventional and complementary medicine are increasingly overlapping, conventional medicine has developed along very different lines to those of the complementary therapies. In conventional medicine, for example, every sign and symptom is said to have a specific cause that can be isolated and treated with a 'formula' such as a drug. Complementary therapies, on the other hand, tend to be holistic and based on the belief that the mind and body are not separate. Practitioners often claim to treat the whole person and to tailor treatments to the individual, and do not just have formulas to hand out for specific symptoms. Here we look at the concepts associated with complementary therapies and assess whether they actually are unique to the field of complementary medicine.

Holism

The holistic approach to health takes the whole person into account – mind, body and spirit – and then tailors treatment to the individual. Many, but not all, complementary therapies purport to take this approach, and have a multifactorial view of ill health and its treatment. They see illness as being due to physical, psychological, social, environmental, spiritual and energetic disturbances, and treat it accordingly. However, some complementary practitioners are 'better' at taking a holistic approach than others; complementary therapists can be narrow and reductionist in their approach. In addition, nowadays, holism is not just practised within the domain of complementary medicine, as more and more doctors are trying to consider their patients as whole people, and many conventional healthcare professionals work in a holistic manner and take a biopsychosocial approach to disease. Furthermore, the ability to listen to and empathise with patients is now being taught in medical schools, and doctors' skills at dealing with patients' emotions and idiosyncrasies are improving. Whoever the practitioner is, the holistic approach is beneficial because it makes people feel more positive if they know someone is taking an interest in them as a person, not just as a medical problem, and is really listening to them.

The mind-body link

The mind-body link is so important to most complementary therapists that they regard it as essential to take the time to explore any psychological factors that might have played a part in causing an illness. Many conventional healthcare practitioners have also recognised for some time that psychological factors influence disease, but they are only now beginning to realise the impact that the mind and emotions can have on the body, and vice versa. In recognition of this, a new field of conventional medicine – psychoneuro-immunology (PNI) – has been flourishing in the USA since the mid-1980s and became established in the UK in the early 1990s.

There is also increasing evidence that the personality of an individual can modify the immune response: for example, people of a cheery, positive disposition may be less likely to become ill than people who are more negative. Research has also shown that stress, particularly severe stress, such as that triggered by bereavement or the breakdown of a marriage, has marked biochemical and hormonal effects within the body. Scientists have shown that complementary therapies that involve relaxation, meditation, hypnotherapy and other psychological interventions may be able to boost the immune system in cancer patients and prolong survival. In addition, several studies have suggested that social support has a significant impact on the survival rate of cancer patients.

'Energy' or vitalism

Many complementary therapies embrace the idea that the body, mind and spirit are all maintained by an underlying 'energy' or vital force. Many practitioners of complementary medicine associate its depletion or imbalance with ill health and its restoration or balance with health. This 'energy' or 'vitalism' is referred to variously as Qi in Traditional Chinese Medicine, prana by Ayurvedic practitioners and yogis, subtle energy by healers, dynamis by homeopaths, vital force by herbalists and osteopaths, innate or universal intelligence by chiropractors and *vis medicatrix naturae* by naturopaths, to name but a few. But what is it? Are the different therapies and therapists all actually referring to the same thing? Does this 'energy' really exist or is it used simply as a metaphor for, or model of, health and illness? Nobody has the answer to these questions yet, although the 'energy' that complementary practitioners refer to is not the same as that referred to in science and conventional medicine, which is concerned with the interconvertibility of matter and energy by living organisms and advocates that energy is solely produced by various cellular metabolic processes. The idea that the body is surrounded and interpenetrated by a more subtle energetic substance is foreign to the 'Western' scientific mind, but many ancient and complementary healing methods refer to a mysterious force we cannot measure with scientific instruments.

The biomedical model that forms the basis of conventional medicine does not seem to have any way of incorporating the concept of 'energy' that is used in complementary medicine. When a patient reports lack of energy it is usually taken to mean physical or mental fatigue and a cause – such as anaemia or hypothyroidism – is searched for. Often no cause can be found. There is no accepted scientific way of measuring, and therefore validating, the level of 'energy' as described in complementary medicine in the human body and so conventional doctors struggle with the concept.

Conventional medicine does measure some energy systems within the body, such as in the heart using an electrocardiograph (ECG) or in the brain using an electroencephalograph (EEG), but this energy is not the same as that referred to in complementary medicine. New computer techniques can now measure the effects of emotions on the autonomic tone of the heart, which in turn reflects the activity in the autonomic nervous system. This has shown that negative emotions such as anger increase the energy in the sympathetic nervous system, while positive emotions such as compassion increase the energy in the parasympathetic nervous system.

The body also gives off thermal or heat energy, as well as sound and light. This electromagnetic energy can now be measured up to a distance of 50cm around the body by means of a sophisticated piece of computer equipment called a magnetometer. A remarkable finding is that the energy given off by the heart is 40–50 times greater than that emitted by the brain, making it the dominant energy source in the body. The energy emitted by the heart flows through every cell in the body, and researchers have now discovered that energy radiating from the heart varies dramatically depending on what sort of mood the patient is in. Scientists have also shown that there may be some sort of energy transfer from one person to another. During experiments to measure the brainwave of one person and the heartbeat of another, they found that when the latter person touched the former, the heartbeat was picked up on the brainwave monitor.

Self-healing, self-regulation and homeostasis

Complementary therapists often say that their aim is to allow or stimulate a person's capacity for self-healing and they largely see their role as providing the right conditions for this to occur and to promote the body's own self-regulating mechanisms. This process of self-regulation is known as homeostasis, that is, good health is the normal, harmonious state for human beings. Disease is generally thought to be due to a lack of harmony. An unhealthy lifestyle and diet can overwhelm the body's natural self-regulating mechanisms and lead to illness. Often the treatment given is aimed at restoring balance and stimulating a self-healing response. Although many conditions do get better by themselves, the idea that the body 'heals itself' is simplistic; for example, when psychosocial factors are a major cause of a mental problem such as depression, simply offering a nutritional supplement is not enough.

Toxins

Some complementary therapists, particularly colonic hydrotherapists (who practise what is popularly known as colonic irrigation), naturopaths, iridologists, some massage therapists as well as aromatherapists, maintain that the human body is full of toxins from the food we eat and the polluted atmosphere in which we live and work. A main aim of some therapists is to rid people of these toxins, although whether toxins are any more than an abstract concept is not clear. It would be foolish to deny that what we eat has an impact on our health, and conventional medicine has long recognised the importance of what we eat. However, a diet that consists of plenty of fresh vegetables and fruit, and moderate amounts of protein and carbohydrates and is low in fat, refined sugars, salt and chemicals is healthy. Fasting and food-exclusion diets can help some conditions (see page 141), but such diets need to be properly supervised.

Patient involvement

Complementary therapists often include advice about lifestyle changes in their treatment, and an attraction can be the support the therapist gives his or her patients while they are trying to make these changes. They might give specific instructions about dietary changes, teach you exercises to do at home, or teach you stress-coping strategies such as relaxation or meditation. Conventional healthcare practitioners are increasingly doing the same, although the complementary therapists' explanations for lifestyle advice might be based on changing body 'energy' or helping the body to heal itself, rather than on a physiological explanation.

Wellness

Many, if not all, complementary therapies embrace the concept of wellness. This is not simply the same as 'not being ill' and is more than the prevention of illness and disease, which is a shared goal by complementary and conventional practitioners alike. It is based more on the concept that, while we may not have any obvious signs and symptoms of ill health, we might not be totally well. Wellness has many facets, ranging from the mental and the spiritual to the physical and even economic level.

Drawbacks of the complementary approach

Complementary medicine appeals to people for various reasons, not all of which may be valid; like any system of treatment, complementary medicine has disadvantages too. The view taken by many therapists – that we are all capable of achieving and maintaining good health, and that we are in a sense responsible for any illness we have – can be problematic as it can lead to feelings of poor self-worth and guilt. This and other unsatisfactory aspects of complementary medicine are discussed below.

Total health

Some complementary practitioners maintain that everyone has the potential to achieve total health by living in as healthy a way as possible, that is, by taking exercise, eating sensibly, not smoking or drinking, and by getting to grips with negative emotions. They believe that all illnesses are caused by an unhealthy lifestyle, an unhealthy environment and negative emotions, all of which are theoretically within our control to change. Some even think that cancer develops as a direct result of repressed anger or a bout of depression. There is no evidence for this, although research suggests that some cancer patients who receive support from friends and family tend to recover faster or at least live longer than those who do not. The goal of total health is in fact misplaced and some people will never be able to attain it, because of their constitution or their genes. In addition, most people develop illness because, by chance, they are infected with a virus or bacteria. Although we are all more susceptible to illness when we are in low spirits, no evidence has shown that being depressed or in an emotional turmoil affects the immune system to the extent that an individual can become seriously ill. However, it is also true that staying fit and eating healthily may well help people ward off colds and flu, as well as illnesses caused by the excesses of modern living.

Individual responsibility

A corollary of the belief that it is in the power of everybody to achieve total health is that a person who is not well is in some way responsible for his or her illness. Some therapists maintain that mental attitudes affect the progress of a disease: if someone is not getting well, it could be because he or she does not have the right attitude to the illness. This, in turn, could make the individual feel guilty, which can hardly be helpful. Another problem with this approach is that it locates the illness and treatment within the individual rather than society: complementary therapists who have these beliefs do not address the issues of inequality and poverty, and the consequent lack of satisfactory housing, inadequate hygiene and poor diet, which are some of the biggest causes of disease. Conventional medicine at least tries to educate people about the importance of a healthy diet and good hygiene.

Antagonism towards conventional medicine

Although reputable complementary therapists would not advise patients to stop taking conventional treatment without consulting their doctors, a few are antagonistic towards conventional medicine and science. Occasionally, people using complementary medicine may themselves share that opinion, and either not visit a GP at all or discontinue medical treatment. Complementary medicine can be extremely harmful if it is used as a substitute for a conventional diagnosis and treatment. Doctors spend years learning not just about anatomy and physiology, but how to diagnose disorders. People may be put at risk by complementary practitioners who are not adequately trained to recognise and manage a disease for which there is a good conventional treatment or who may make a wrong diagnosis.

'Natural' equals 'safe'

Complementary medicine is popular partly because it is seen as natural and non-invasive, but believing that a therapy is good for you merely because it is 'natural' can be unwise. It is true that complementary remedies are made from naturally occurring plants and oils, which are generally regarded as safe when compared with the synthetic, laboratory-produced chemicals used in mainstream treatments; also, they have few unpleasant side-effects. However, natural substances are not always safe; deadly nightshade, rhubarb leaves and uncooked kidney beans can be extremely toxic, as can a few berries and mushrooms. Some herbal remedies have been found to contain poisons or to be contaminated with conventional medicines (see page 115). Nevertheless, the number of people who have died as a direct result of taking complementary medicines is low compared with the number of deaths associated with conventional medicines. There are also rare risks associated with some of the therapies if used inappropriately, such as injury from spinal manipulation or infection from acupuncture.

To say that only 'natural' treatments are beneficial can be equally wrong and dangerous. Scientists have spent years developing many successful life-saving drugs and techniques. In many cases, synthetic drugs are more effective than complementary treatments.

'Ancient' equals 'good'

The fact that many complementary therapies have their roots in ancient practices, for example, from Egypt, India, China and Japan, and have therefore stood the test of time, also attracts people to them. 'Old', like 'natural', is often thought to mean 'good'. Although some ancient treatments do have merit (for example, t'ai chi is calming and acupuncture relieves pain), others, such as blood-letting, are completely ineffective and can be dangerous. There is no reason why an ancient therapy should, per se, be more effective or better for you than a modern one.

Chapter 2

Who uses complementary therapies, and why?

Complementary therapies are more popular in the UK today than ever before, with an estimated 4–5 million people seeing a complementary therapist each year. The reasons for the increase in acceptability and use of such therapies reveal a great deal about social trends in the latter part of the twentieth century. This chapter explores the history of the growth in the complementary medicine field and looks at the kinds of people who use complementary therapies and why.

Even as recently as the 1960s complementary medicine was a fringe interest in the UK; before that there was not even a general name by which these therapies were known. It was not until the 1980s that interest really started growing, not only from patients and the general public but also from doctors and other healthcare professionals.

The reasons why people turn to complementary medicine are both negative (such as disillusionment with certain aspects of conventional medicine) and positive (the fact that so many people claim to have benefited from it). Nevertheless, research suggests that most people tend to use complementary therapies alongside conventional medicine, rather than as an alternative to it, sometimes for different complaints, sometimes together for the same complaint.

The growth in complementary medicine

One study conducted in England in 1993 found that about 8.5 per cent of the adult population had received at least one of the following main complementary therapies in the previous year: acupuncture, chiropractic, homeopathy, hypnotherapy, herbal medicine or osteopathy. Five years later, a similar study found that this had increased to 10.6 per cent. In a more recent study, around 25 per cent of the public said they had used one of the main six therapies, which rose to 33 per cent when aromatherapy and reflexology were added. In another UK survey, in 1999, an estimated 20 per cent of people had used some type of complementary therapy or bought an over-the-counter remedy in the previous 12 months.

In a survey conducted by Consumers' Association in 1995, nearly 9,000 subscribers to *Which?* responded, and almost one in three reported having used complementary medicine at some time in their lives. Of those who had used it, one in five had done so during the preceding year, and women were more likely to have tried it than men (40 per cent versus 27 per cent). The *Which?* survey also found that an increasing proportion of young, fit people are turning to complementary medicine. Although some people (41 per cent) said that they had used complementary medicine to alleviate a long-term condition, many reported using it to maintain and enhance their health.

Other polls have shown that people living in the south of England visit more complementary practitioners than those living in the north and Scotland, and that complementary therapy is most popular in the west of England. Research has also shown that most people who use complementary medicine are adults, aged between of 21 and 60 years, and that, while people from all social classes consult complementary therapists, those from higher socio-economic groups are more likely to do so. This is presumably because they have the necessary disposable income, given that complementary therapies are predominantly used in the private paying sector. A survey in the late 1980s found that 74 per cent of the UK population said they would use complementary therapies if they were widely available on the National Health Service (NHS).

Several studies have found that problems with the muscles and joints are by far the most common reason for using complementary medicine, accounting for around 60 per cent of consultations. In the private sector, patients most commonly have complementary therapy for long-term, painful, mild to moderate problems that are often stress-related and cause problems with function rather than measurable pathophysiological changes. Most of them have already tried conventional treatment for their condition. Surveys also suggest, however, that people with chronic and difficult to manage diseases, such as arthritic and rheumatic conditions, cancer, HIV infection, psoriasis and multiple sclerosis, are twice as likely to consult a complementary therapist as people with other conditions.

Among the most popular complementary therapies are acupuncture, chiropractic, herbal medicine, homeopathy and osteopathy, with healing and hypnotherapy also frequently mentioned. Also, as many as a third of people in the UK use complementary self-help techniques and remedies, such as meditation, relaxation, herbs and supplements.

Why the increase in popularity?

There are probably many reasons why complementary therapies have increased in popularity. Up until the late 1960s, people still had complete faith in conventional medicine; doctors were respected members of the post-war community, and they had the time to talk to and visit their patients. Old-fashioned practices, such as herbal medicine and homeopathy, were tolerated, partly perhaps because the royal family and upper classes favoured them, but therapies new to the West, such as acupuncture, were viewed as suspect.

A substantial shift in attitudes has taken place since then. This has, in part, been due to a growing disillusionment with conventional medicine and many of its approaches to treatment, and may also be partly due to the desire for more equal relationships between patients and healthcare providers that is embodied in the new consumerism of today.

Despite the promises of the 1950s and '60s, medicine has often failed to deal successfully with many chronic conditions, such as arthritis and eczema, and cures for common illnesses such as colds and flu still do not exist. Moreover, some of the side-effects resulting from taking conventional medicines are nasty and even dangerous, and are often a reason why people turn to complementary medicine. For example, up to 2,000 people are believed to die each year in the UK alone from severe stomach bleeding due to nonsteroidal anti-inflammatory drugs (NSAIDs) taken to relieve the pain and inflammation of arthritis. Another source of dissatisfaction has been the long waiting time for hospital treatment in the overstretched National Health Service, and the lack of time with the doctor once you get to see one.

It is not just the type of treatment by practitioners of conventional medicine that people are unhappy with; it is their approach as well. Conventional medicine has developed along paternalistic, reductionist and mechanistic lines. Doctors have been seen as all-knowing and patients have been expected to comply with what they are told to do and not ask questions. Every sign and symptom of disease is believed to have a specific cause, which can be treated by targeting the specific part(s) of the body affected, usually using drugs or surgery.

Finally, some people do turn to complementary therapies because of a total rejection of conventional medicine due to anti-scientific or anti-establishment attitudes.

Complementary medicine has several perceived advantages over conventional medicine, which influence why people turn to it. These include: the holistic approach (see page 18) believed to be taken by complementary therapists, who claim to recognise that the mind and body influence each other strongly; the self-help aspect of many complementary therapies, that encourages and helps people to take control of their health; the relationship with the therapist, who has the time and willingness for discussion with the patient, and does so on an equal footing; and a belief in the philosophical basis of the therapy chosen. Some research in the USA suggests that it is philosophical congruence that is most predictive of complementary therapy use and that, rather than turning to complementary medicine because of disillusionment with conventional medicine, people are most likely to be drawn to a complementary therapy because it is seen as more compatible with their philosophies or beliefs about health and illness, their values and their world view. The features that people seem to find resonance with include the assumed association of complementary therapies with 'energy', 'nature' and 'spirituality'.

Complementary therapies worldwide

The popularity of complementary therapies is not confined to the UK; indeed, consumers in many other Western countries spend more than those in the UK on natural remedies and complementary therapies. Results from a telephone survey in 1990 suggest that Americans made 425 million visits to complementary practitioners in that year, compared with 388 million visits to primary-care physicians (a category that includes GPs but not hospital doctors), and an estimated 42 per cent of people in the USA used a complementary therapy in 1997.

Results from a study in 1993 showed that 49 per cent of Australians used complementary therapies, spending a total of A$930 million on visiting complementary therapists and consuming natural remedies, while a survey published in 1996 in Australia revealed that one in five Australians regularly visits a complementary practitioner. In Australia, acupuncture is the most popular complementary therapy, while in New Zealand, about one in four GPs uses acupuncture.

In France, around 48 per cent of people regularly visit a complementary therapist; in Germany it is about 46 per cent; in Belgium 31 per cent; and in the Netherlands 20 per cent. National preferences vary: for example, massage is very popular in Finland, the Dutch are keen on spiritual healers, and in Germany and France homeopathy is particularly popular.

Chapter 3

Complementary therapy providers

The growth in popularity of complementary medicine in the UK is reflected in the rapid increase in registered complementary therapists; from 1981 to 1997, the number of non-medically qualified registered practitioners trebled from around 13,500 to about 50,000. Alongside this, there has also been an increase in medically qualified healthcare practitioners who are now practising complementary therapies within the conventional medical setting. A recent development is the notion of 'integrated healthcare', combining complementary and conventional medicine, which is gaining interest in many circles.

Who provides complementary therapies?

Most complementary therapies are provided by non-medically qualified practitioners. Of the estimated 50,000 registered practitioners now practising in the UK, the largest group are healers (about 14,000), with aromatherapists (7,000) and reflexologists (5,000) the second and third largest groups. However, few complementary therapists practise full time, except perhaps chiropractors and osteopaths. Several thousand conventional healthcare professionals also practise some form or other of complementary medicine and are registered with their own organisation, such as the British Medical Acupuncture Society* or the Faculty of Homeopathy*. Of these, around 50 per cent (mainly doctors and physiotherapists) practise acupuncture, about 25 per cent (mainly nurses) practise reflexology and massage and about 15 per cent (mainly doctors, and podiatrists and chiropodists) practise homeopathy. Many more conventional healthcare professionals are not officially registered as complementary therapists but offer limited complementary techniques that they have learnt on basic or introductory courses.

Complementary therapies in the NHS

Complementary therapies are mainly provided via the private sector, either paid for out of one's own pocket or through private health insurance, but over the past 15 years there has been a significant increase in the amount of complementary medicine being accessed via the NHS. While homeopathy has been available under the NHS at five hospitals since 1948, other complementary therapies have become available under the NHS only since the late 1980s. This was, in part, due to a highly critical report published in 1986 by the British Medical Association (BMA)* entitled *Alternative therapy*, in which many therapies were dismissed as being untested, ineffective and potentially harmful. They were, it concluded, based on 'primitive beliefs and outmoded practices, almost all without basis', and their popularity was attributed to both the irrationality of consumers and the failure of doctors to address the wider needs of their patients. Seven years later, however, the BMA produced *Complementary medicine: new approaches to good practice*. In it, complementary medicine was referred to as 'non-conventional therapies', and the tone of the report was noticeably more balanced and conciliatory. The BMA had accepted that complementary medicine was more than just a passing phase, and decided to work with it. In addition, in December 1991, the Department of Health acknowledged the public demand for NHS access to complementary medicine by giving family doctors the go-ahead to employ complementary practitioners as ancillary staff, provided that the GPs retained clinical responsibility, or to use complementary medicine themselves for treating patients.

In addition, patients seem happy with the complementary therapies they receive through the NHS. In 2001, researchers at the University of Sheffield interviewed 49 NHS patients at eight general practices and found that their views about the treatments they had received were overwhelmingly positive. They all reported that the complementary therapies they had received had helped to relieve or cure their symptoms, including chronic problems. The patients had also found the practitioners to be calm and caring and had liked the way they were encouraged to take an active part in their own healthcare. Very few had any complaints. The researchers concluded that the patients had been satisfied regardless of the setting or type of therapy they had received. They also found that the patients' satisfaction with their treatment was mainly due to the positive experience rather than any prior positive beliefs about the therapy they received.

Complementary medicine in primary care

According to a study carried out by the University of Sheffield for the Department of Health in 1995, around four in ten GPs in England then provided access to some form of complementary therapy for their NHS patients. The study found that, in one week, 45 per cent of GPs recommended or endorsed the use of complementary therapies in their consultations, 21 per cent referred patients to a complementary therapist, both privately and under the NHS, six per cent employed an 'independent' complementary therapist, and one in ten GPs treated patients with a complementary therapy themselves.

However, according to a report by the Foundation for Integrated Medicine (FIM)★, which analysed Primary Care Group (PCG) plans for complementary medicine from 1999 to 2000, the abolition of GP fundholding and the advent of PCGs has had a dramatic effect on the provision of complementary medicine on the NHS. It found that many therapies previously paid for out of GP fundholders' budgets were cut completely. The reasons for this included lack of evidence to support their use, or lack of equal access because the therapies provided were not available across the whole PCG. However, some PCGs have seen the new arrangements as an opportunity to ensure equality exists by extending provision of complementary medicine across the whole PCG. As more PCGs become Primary Care Trusts (PCTs), with control over their own budgets, there could be more opportunity for complementary medicine in primary care, and there are some signs that this is going to be the case. A study (published in 2000) of complementary therapy provision in PCGs, which involved sending out a questionnaire to all 481 PCGs, found that more than half of the 60 per cent who responded said that some form of complementary medicine was provided within its area. The most commonly used therapies were acupuncture, osteopathy, chiropractic, homeopathy and hypnotherapy. A survey carried out by the University of Westminster in 2001 of the 32 PCGs and PCTs in London found that two-thirds offered complementary medicine services, with the most popular therapies being acupuncture, osteopathy, homeopathy and therapeutic massage.

Complementary therapies in hospitals

About 65 per cent of British hospital doctors think that complementary medicine has a place in mainstream medicine. Although not many hospitals explicitly offer complementary medicine, many nurses routinely incorporate it into their nursing practices; in particular, massage, aromatherapy and reflexology are being used increasingly. Nurses are in fact among the main players in the expansion of complementary therapy in NHS hospitals. The Royal College of Nursing has a Complementary Therapies Nursing Forum, with over 2,000 members, and nurses have spearheaded some 80 per cent of cases where policies for the practice of complementary therapies are being or have been developed in health services around Britain. Other complementary medicine provision within secondary care includes: acupuncture in pain clinics (given by anaesthetists, physiotherapists or palliative care physicians); yoga and acupuncture in obstetrics departments (by midwives or physiotherapists); and acupuncture and manipulative therapy in rheumatology and physiotherapy departments (by chiropractors, osteopaths, physiotherapists or orthopaedic physicians).

Complementary medicine in other settings

Health authorities are beginning to fund the use of complementary therapies in sheltered accommodation and residential homes for older people, and in Community Drug and Alcohol Units. Hospices are also big providers of complementary medicine. One survey of 18 hospices in England found that all of them offered aromatherapy and massage, 81 per cent offered reflexology, 31 per cent acupuncture, 25 per cent reiki and 37 per cent other therapies such as hypnotherapy and shiatsu. There are also schemes, such as the one funded by Camden Social Services department in London, that are taking complementary therapies into the community. In conjunction with the charity Women and Health, Camden Social

Services runs Care in the Community Schemes whereby women caring for a relation with mental illness or children with disabilities can have a course of one of a variety of complementary therapies in their own homes.

Integrated healthcare

Recent research has found that there is growing interest in integrating complementary therapies into primary care, with as many as one in ten Primary Care Trusts (PCTs) seeking to establish PCT-wide complementary and alternative medicine services. Integrated services are also being established in Health Action Zones, Healthy Living Centres and other initiatives set up by the government to combat health inequalities, often in conjunction with PCT partners, and taking referrals from local GPs.

The Foundation for Integrated Medicine★ has established a new integrated healthcare collaborative for people setting up and running integrated healthcare services, that is, services that provide complementary and alternative therapies alongside more conventional healthcare provision in primary care settings. The initiative involves the establishment of a learning collaborative and, in partnership with the University of Westminster in London, a support and information network. Its aims are to: support joint learning between a set of projects representing different models of integrated primary care provision; explore different strategies for the development of integrated projects within primary care organisations and find out what steps and resources are required; develop resources that can be used by others seeking to develop integrated primary care elsewhere (particularly information and knowledge resources); gather evidence about successful models and development strategies; share the learning from this work with a wider network of people.

The Foundation is providing support to the projects taking part in the collaborative in a number of ways, including: funding (up to £5,000) for participation in the collaborative seminars; funding (up to £5,000) towards the costs of development activities and their evaluation; expert advice on service development, models of integrated working and evaluation strategies; information, for example, about possible sources of funding; and relevant research on effectiveness and cost–effectiveness of complementary therapy in primary care.

Chapter 4

Finding a reliable practitioner

In the UK, there is little direct regulation of non-medically qualified complementary practitioners; until relatively recently, under common law, all complementary therapists could practise freely and do more or less what they wanted, subject only to minor legislation. However, recent Acts of Parliament have established the General Chiropractic Council (GCC)★ and the General Osteopathic Council (GosC)★ for the statutory self-regulation of these professions and now, only practitioners registered with these bodies may use the titles Chiropractor and Osteopath, respectively. Acupuncture, herbal medicine and homeopathy are likely to follow suit in the next few years. But, until then, anyone, regardless of qualifications or experience, can set him- or herself up as any type of complementary therapist (other than a chiropractor or osteopath). The only legislation there is forbids non-medically qualified practitioners from claiming to be a state-registered professional, such as a dentist, doctor or physiotherapist (and now an osteopath or chiropractor), or to be able to cure certain medical conditions, such as cancer, diabetes, epilepsy, tuberculosis and venereal disease. In this chapter, we look at how you can find an appropriately qualified practitioner, and what you can do if you are dissatisfied with a treatment you have received.

Although complementary medicine generally appears to be far safer than conventional medicine, it does carry risks, with thousands of adverse effects from complementary therapies being reported worldwide, including well over 100 deaths. The highest risk probably comes from unqualified practitioners. However, most complementary therapies have registering bodies, through which you can find out more about the therapy and check that the person you are thinking of consulting is fully qualified in his or her field. Information about these bodies is in Parts II and III, under the relevant therapies, and contact details are given in the Addresses section.

Regulation of complementary medicine

Most complementary therapies are regulated by one or more voluntary body and the way they are run varies from therapy to therapy. Without proper legislation and protection of title within the field of complementary medicine, the consumer is likely always to be short-changed. Ideally, each complementary therapy should have a single registering body, and consumers should be able to trust a practitioner's registration with such a body as proof that they are reputable. Indeed, increasingly, practitioners have grown to realise that if they are to continue enjoying the common-law freedom to practise that characterises complementary medicine in the UK they must put their house in order. Much more emphasis is now being placed on standardising, accrediting and validating training courses with an organisation that the public can see is *bona fide* and that has codes of practice and ethics. Continuing professional development is also becoming a requirement with many organisations.

One of the recommendations in the report on Complementary and Alternative Medicine by the House of Lords Select Committee on Science and Technology was 'that only those CAM therapies which are statutorily regulated, or have a powerful mechanism of voluntary self-regulation, should be made available by reference from doctors and other healthcare professionals working in primary, secondary or tertiary care, on the NHS'. They also concluded that better regulation of complementary and alternative medicine is essential to protect the needs of patients and the public. In their view, this meant, as a first step, the development of single voluntary regulatory bodies for each therapy. For two professions, herbal medicine and acupuncture, plus possibly homeopathy in the future, they also recommended statutory regulation on a similar basis to chiropractic and osteopathy. Their criteria for recommending statutory regulation were: the possible risk to the public from poor practice; a pre-existing robust voluntary regulatory system; and the presence of a credible evidence base. The enquiry also concluded that, in the absence of clear guidelines for regulation and training of statutory practitioners, such as doctors and nurses, who incorporate CAM therapies into their medical practice, the relevant regulatory body, for example the General Medical Council (GMC)*, should develop clear guidelines on competency and training for its members.

In its published response to the report, the government accepted virtually all of the report's recommendations. It also stated that complementary medicine has a role to play within the NHS but must meet the same standards as other NHS treatments, must be clear and realistic about the contributions it can make, and that preliminary changes within complementary therapy professions should now be driven forward more decisively. What the response was not explicit about is what funding, if any, will be made available to help drive these changes forward.

In the meantime, because changes are happening very slowly, the consumer is often faced with a bewildering number of registering bodies for each therapy. Many have impressive-sounding names, such as the International Association of X or the British Council for Y, but there are no official guidelines as to which ones are genuine and which ones are 'better' than others.

Safeguards

The best organisations will have the following safeguards:

1. **A set of validated, and accredited, educational and training standards**. More and more organisations are realising the importance of good training in order to ensure that their members are fit to practice, and have developed minimum requirements for education and training that have been accredited and standardised.
2. **A code of practice and ethics** that at least covers: the legal obligations of practitioners; the treatment limitations that a particular therapy can offer or claim to offer; expected professional conduct towards patients; how therapists should relate to medical practitioners; and what kind of information should be given and what claims should not be made to patients. It should include requirements to: keep good records; preserve patient confidentiality; have decent premises; advertise services and fees in a reasonable fashion; and deal with patients' complaints properly.

3. **A complaints procedure**. The best complaints procedures are accessible, fair and effective. They should be well-publicised and free for complainants to use. Complaints should be easy to make and should be dealt with as swiftly as possible.

4. **Disciplinary procedures**, such as suspension or removal of the practitioner from the register. Disciplinary procedures should be open, and it should be clear that practitioners can be disciplined if they fail to comply with the code of practice and ethics.

5. **A requirement for indemnity insurance**, against malpractice or negligence claims.

However, while most registering bodies do have elaborate codes of practice and ethics, and if a practitioner fails to abide by them he or she can be struck off, this is not comparable to a doctor being struck off by the GMC. This is because medicine is regulated by the state, and a doctor has to register with the GMC before he or she can practise. If, subsequently, a complaint is made against that doctor and he or she is found guilty of serious professional misconduct, the GMC's ultimate sanction would be to have that doctor struck off and his or her name erased from the register. It would then be a criminal offence for that doctor to practise within the NHS and write out NHS prescriptions (although he or she could still write out private prescriptions), and if such a doctor were found practising he or she would be prosecuted. This is also now true for chiropractors and osteopaths. Being 'struck off' is not as serious for other complementary practitioners, who, having been ousted from a particular association one week, could easily join another organisation the following week and open for business again legally.

Umbrella organisations representing complementary medicine

The growth of complementary therapies has prompted the formation of several umbrella organisations, founded between 1981 and 1990. These primarily represent the interests of practitioners, which may not necessarily be the same as those of consumers. Two main umbrella organisations have been established, as well as various campaigning groups.

The **British Complementary Medicine Association (BCMA)**⋆ was set up in 1990 and is the largest overall body, and claims to represent about 25,000 practitioners in 67 organisations covering 30 therapies. Its stated aim is to encourage the diverse organisations of individual therapies to join together into single therapy groups and act collectively. It is the organisations, not the individuals who belong to them, that pay to be on the register the BCMA runs. Members of the public can contact the BCMA either to check on the qualifications of a practitioner or to find a qualified therapist in a particular field who practises in their area. Each therapy belongs to a 'therapy group' within the BCMA, which dictates what training and qualifications are needed for membership, and practitioners must fulfil the criteria laid down by the group. It also has published codes of ethics, conduct and disciplinary procedures. The BCMA is a non-profit-making organisation. Its committee members are elected annually and are unpaid, so they claim that the BCMA is more independent than the Institute of Complementary Medicine, which is run by two paid directors. The **Institute for Complementary Medicine (ICM)**★ was established as a charity in 1982 to provide information for the public about complementary practitioners. It claims to represents about 2,000 practitioners in nearly 800 organisations covering approximately 18 therapies on its British Register of Complementary Practitioners (BRCP).

In addition, the **Council for Complementary and Alternative Medicine (CCAM)**★ provides a forum for communication and co-operation between professional bodies representing acupuncture, herbal medicine, homeopathy, naturopathy and osteopathy. It was set up to support the professional development of these five disciplines and to promote public knowledge of good-quality complementary care. The **Natural Medicines Society (NMS)**★ was set up in 1985 to protect consumers' right to have access to high-quality alternative treatment and it works to ensure that natural medicines are safe and produced to a high standard. Claiming that complementary medicine is still under threat, it has embarked on a campaign to safeguard such medicine from 'ill-informed interference' and to push for high standards of training. To this end, it has set up a Medicines Advisory Research Committee, which can be called upon by government bodies for advice. Both the CCAM and the NMS lobby on behalf of complementary therapies when these are threatened by adverse legislation.

Both have close links with the All-Party Parliamentary Group for Alternative and Complementary Medicine and have occasional meetings with ministers. This active parliamentary group is a forum for the exchange of views promoting 'sensible' policies on complementary medicine.

The **Foundation for Integrated Medicine (FIM)**★ was established in the UK in 1997, as a result of an initiative by the Prince of Wales. Its aim is to promote the development and integrated delivery of safe, effective and efficient forms of healthcare, including conventional and complementary medicine, to patients and their families by encouraging greater collaboration between all forms of healthcare. A similar body, the National Center for Complementary and Alternative Medicine (NCCAM)★, has been established in the USA. It is essentially an agency which funds research in complementary medicine, and now receives $100 million a year to plough into the area.

Complementary therapies and the European Community

There are huge national variations in the regulation of complementary therapies, the law, market forces, medical attitude, state funding, health beliefs and practices within the European Community.

The UK is fortunate in that consumers have widespread access to complementary systems of medicine that several other European citizens do not have, such as herbalism, homeopathy and acupuncture. In some member states of the EU, including France, Spain, Italy and Greece, it is illegal for anyone except statutorily recognised health professionals to practise medicine; this includes all non-medically qualified complementary practitioners. In France and Spain, the authorities are particularly tough on clamping down on non-medically qualified complementary practitioners. However, in the Netherlands the government has stated that it will not prosecute non-medically qualified practitioners unless malpractice has been proven; complementary therapies are generally tolerated by the Dutch authorities and in fact flourish. In Germany, the unique *Heilpraktiker* (health system) was introduced in 1939. It licenses practitioners who are not members of recognised health professions to practise complementary medicine provided they are registered. In Belgium, the government has recently paved the way for the formal recognition of four types of complementary medicine: acupuncture, chiropractic, homeopathy and osteopathy.

A proposal on complementary medicine drafted by the Belgian Green MEP Paul Lannoye was presented to the European Union Committee on the Environment, Public Health and Consumer Protection in April 1996. The report called for freedom for consumers in Europe to choose what type of treatment they want, while appropriate guarantees for their safety are ensured. These guarantees could be obtained through higher standards of training for practitioners, which should be harmonised throughout the EU, and through high-quality manufacturing procedures for all healthcare products. This would mean the establishment of recognised professional bodies for each individual complementary therapy in each member state, similar to the UK's General Osteopathic Council (GOsC)*, although, unlike the GOsC, the bodies concerned would not have to be enshrined in statute. Such a structure would allow for mutual recognition between member states, the free movement of appropriately qualified therapists around Europe, and a wider choice of treatment options for all European citizens.

In February 2002, the European Commission made formal proposals for a European-wide Directive on traditional herbal medicinal products. The proposals aim to introduce specific requirements for the safety and quality of over-the-counter medicines made from herbal ingredients. Unlike the requirement for proof of efficacy needed to license a conventional medicine, proof of a history of traditional use will be required (probably evidence that the product has been on the market for at least 30 years, including 15 years in Europe), along with a statement on packaging that the medicine's efficacy is not proven. While this should make for safer herbal medicines, which is a welcome move, it could also mean that newer products, and ancient products from other cultures that have been used in Europe only for a short while, may not qualify, and so could, in effect, become unavailable. A new European Directive on Food Supplements containing vitamins and minerals was imminent as this book went to press. The Directive contains a list of nutrients that may be used in food supplements, but at present, there are several nutrients on the UK market that are not included in the list. It also gives maximum limits for the dosages allowed in food supplements, which are lower than those in many currently available supplements.

Choosing a therapy and a therapist

Deciding whether to opt for a complementary therapy, and choosing which one is best for you, can be daunting, especially given the number of therapies available and the differences between them. Even before considering the pros and cons of individual therapies, it is worth asking yourself why you want to use complementary medicine. Is it for the treatment of an existing ailment or for maintaining good health? If it is for the former, think carefully about whether your expectations are realistic: are you looking to complementary medicine to cure the ailment or to alleviate the symptoms and help you live with it? Do you want to try complementary medicine because you are dissatisfied with conventional medicine? Or, is it because specific aspects of complementary medicine attract you to it? Whatever your reasons for wanting to try complementary medicine, if you have an existing condition or symptoms of an illness, it is a good idea to consult your GP before embarking upon any therapy.

Many ailments and conditions can be helped by more than one therapy. For example, migraine can be treated by acupuncture, herbal medicine or relaxation therapy, while back pain can be treated by chiropractic, osteopathy, massage, the Alexander technique, yoga, herbal medicine or acupuncture. Of the therapies that seem most relevant to your needs, choose the one (or more) that appeals to you most in terms of its philosophy and technique. You may, for example, find the Traditional Chinese Medical way of explaining ill health in terms of blockages of Qi (energy) a satisfactory one, but may have a fear of needles, which would rule out acupuncture. The likely cost of a therapy and the availability in your area of a suitably qualified practitioner are also important considerations. Be prepared to commit yourself to a full course of treatment, and also to stop having it if, after a while, you feel it is not helpful.

It is often possible to combine therapies; indeed, many practitioners themselves use a range of therapeutic techniques to treat people. Naturopaths, for instance, are often also trained in several other therapies, such as osteopathy or homeopathy, some acupuncturists are also trained in Chinese herbalism and many Ayurvedic practitioners could, as well as prescribing you herbs, use massage or yoga to treat you. If you choose to use different therapies from different practitioners at the same time ensure that the individual practitioners know about it.

If you do want to try a complementary therapy, your best chance of being satisfied is to find a well-trained, reputable practitioner. It is vital that you check out the therapist's credentials, and it is also important to choose a practitioner you feel comfortable with. Personal recommendation can be a good way of finding such a therapist, but not always. A friend or colleague may have built up a rapport with a particular therapist, but you may not be able to do so. If you have already decided which therapy you want to try, then you could contact the relevant registering body (or bodies), as some of them will supply you with a list of qualified practitioners in your area. You could also take advice from your GP, but he or she may be unenthusiastic about complementary therapies as a whole, or may be no better informed about them than you are. Many well-qualified practitioners advertise in *Yellow Pages,* in the same way that opticians, dentists and doctors do, but remember that anyone can be listed. Your local natural healing centre could be a good source of the names of local practitioners and the staff should be able to suggest which therapy might suit you. It is inadvisable, however, to look for therapists at natural healing fairs and festivals, in advertisements displayed in libraries and newsagents, or via a mail-shot through your door. Also, regard anyone who approaches you directly, in person or by phone, with suspicion: reputable practitioners do not hawk for business. Never be fooled by glossy brochures and impressive-looking credentials either. Practitioners' diplomas and licences are not always genuine, and even if they are, they may be of little or no value. Remember, if anything about a therapist sounds too good to be true, it probably is!

Whatever way you find a therapist, always check the practitioner's qualifications with the organisation to which he or she claims to belong. However, even membership of an organisation is no guarantee of quality and good practice – you still need to check out the professional organisation itself. Some organisations are interested only in collecting the registration fee and have little or no idea of the quality and experience of the people on their books. Choosing a therapist who belongs to a reputable professional organisation is vital.

Once you have found a practitioner you are considering seeing, it is advisable to talk to him or her before you book an appointment. A good practitioner, far from objecting to your questions, will probably welcome them. If he or she refuses to answer them, look for another practitioner. Ask yourself whether: the practitioner seems warm, genuine, caring, sympathetic and trustworthy; whether you will be able to confide in him or her; and whether he or she seems hopeful about treating you.

Picking the right therapist ultimately depends on personal choice. You may, for example, prefer a practitioner of the same gender as yourself for therapies such as massage and osteopathy, where close physical contact is necessary. If you have a chronic condition, it may be that you will see the therapist once a month or once every two months for many years, so it is important to have a good relationship with that person; forming a positive relationship with a therapist may improve your chances of recovery.

Questions to ask a potential practitioner

- What are your methods of treatment? Are they appropriate to my condition?
- How does the process work?
- What sort of person does (or does not) benefit from the treatment?
- How many sessions might I need before I see any improvement?
- What are your qualifications and how long did you train for?
- How long have you been practising?
- To which professional body do you belong?
- Are you covered by professional indemnity insurance?
- How much will the treatment cost?

A good practitioner will ...

- welcome any questions you have and answer them fully
- give a full explanation of all the procedures involved in the treatment and tell you how you may feel afterwards
- tell you how much treatment will cost and give you a rough estimate of how many treatment sessions you may need to have
- have had adequate training, not have trained through a correspondence course, and belong to a recognised organisation
- not guarantee recovery and will tell you if he or she cannot help you
- have full professional indemnity insurance
- not over-charge.

A bad practitioner will ...

- be rude, arrogant or offended when you ask questions
- promise to cure your condition (responsible practitioners, on the other hand, know that a cure cannot be guaranteed and that no medicine or therapy is 100 per cent effective)
- promise cures for specific conditions (responsible practitioners will say no more than that the treatment they are administering is sometimes successful in cases such as yours)
- tell you to stop seeing your doctor and/or to stop taking your medication
- not listen to you or take a full case history – or, conversely, take a prying, salacious interest in your personal life
- not take notes
- rubbish the work of other therapists and doctors
- make you feel uneasy or uncomfortable
- tell you a lot of mumbo-jumbo
- charge far more (or far less) than other practitioners.

Complaining about a practitioner

Most people who visit a complementary practitioner are happy with their treatment. In a survey published in *Which?* in December 2001, which involved sending questionnaires to about 10,000 *Which?* and *Health Which?* members to find out how helpful they had found complementary therapies, only 3 per cent of the 1,198 people who responded said that they wanted to complain about a therapist. In total, 2 per cent of them went on to do so. The main problems that people were unhappy about were a lack of improvement in their condition, feeling worse due to the therapy, poor service, side-effects and the cost of treatment.

If you feel you have been short-changed, either financially or in terms of the treatment you have received, you have several options.

1. You can in the first instance complain directly to the practitioner. Talk or write to him or her about what happened (keep a copy of the letter). It may be that you have experienced a temporary adverse reaction that occurs commonly after the type of treatment you have undergone.
2. If you get no response from the practitioner and you want to take the matter further, complain in writing to the professional or

regulatory body of which he or she is a member. Most such bodies have complaints procedures and codes of practice and ethics. The practitioner will usually be invited to respond, and a committee will decide what action should be taken.

3. Complain in writing to the umbrella organisation, such as the BCMA★ or ICM★, to which the therapist belongs. These bodies also have codes of conduct and can deal with complaints.

4. If the practitioner is employed in a health centre or sports centre, complain in writing to its manager.

5. If the practitioner is employed by the NHS, you see him or her on an NHS basis, or you have been referred by your GP and are not happy with the treatment you have received, you should in the first instance complain to the practitioner, then to your GP. If you subsequently feel you have not received a satisfactory reply or explanation, complain to the senior partner in the GP practice. If you had treatment under the NHS in a hospital, which you consider unsatisfactory, complain in writing to the chief executive; your letter will be passed on to the complaints or customer services manager. You can also use the statutory NHS complaints procedure. This is a two-stage process comprising local and a possible 'independent' review within local NHS Trusts or health authorities. If the NHS complaints procedure does not result in a satisfactory result, you can complain to the Health Service Commissioner (or Ombudsman)★.

If despite following this guidance you are still unhappy, you may wish to resort to the legal system (see Chapter 5).

Chapter 5

Complementary medicine and the law

The practice of medicine in the UK is regulated by various Acts passed since the time of the Tudors and Stuarts. The Medical Act 1512 was the first to attempt to regulate the profession, and made it an 'offence to practise physic or surgery' unless the practitioner was a university graduate or had been licensed by the bishop of the diocese in which he lived. This legislation was not popular, and as a result of public opinion the king was forced to amend the Act in 1542 to allow anyone to practise. This has become known as the Herbalists' Charter.

The Herbalists' Charter

This Act, which had the support of Henry VIII, was designed to help those people who could not afford the increasingly avaricious surgeons and physicians who allowed the sick 'to rot and perish to death' unless they could pay. The legislation made it lawful for anyone who had knowledge and experience of the nature of 'Herbs, roots and Waters ... to practise, use and minister in and to any outward sore, uncome, wound, apostemations, outward swelling or disease, any herb or herbs, oyntments, baths, pultres and amplaisters, according to their cunning, experience and knowledge ... without suit, vexation, trouble, penalty, or loss of their goods'. This right to practise freely and legally is guarded jealously by herbalists and supported by the government. Herbalists are still under no obligation to clear what they prescribe with the Medicines Control Agency★ (the government regulatory body for medicines). Four hundred years later the Herbal Remedies Order 1977 defined the circumstances under which herbalists could prescribe certain toxic herbs, such as belladonna.

The Medical Act of 1858

The Medical Act of 1858 made it illegal for anyone who had not been registered as a qualified medical practitioner to claim to be one. It empowered the General Medical Council (GMC)★ to oversee the regulation and training of the medical profession. However, it did not prohibit non-orthodox or non-registered practitioners from treating patients, providing they did not claim to be registered doctors. It also allowed qualified doctors to administer non-orthodox medical treatments if they so wished, as long as they adhered to professional standards of care. Such standards are established in law using the 'Bolam test', which states that 'a doctor is not guilty of negligence if he or she has acted in accordance with a practice accepted as proper by a responsible body of medical men skilled in that particular art as long as it is subject to logical analysis'. This means that doctors can justify using a complementary treatment if they have undertaken some sort of training in it, and that their use of the treatment is considered acceptable by a number (not necessarily a majority) of other medically qualified users of the complementary treatment.

Doctors cannot 'refer' you to a complementary practitioner in the same way that they can refer you to a hospital consultant. When a doctor refers you to another specialist, that specialist takes responsibility for your treatment, and takes the blame if anything goes wrong. When a doctor refers you for a complementary therapy, he or she 'delegates' your treatment to the complementary practitioner. This means that doctors remain responsible for the negligence of any complementary practitioner who is employed on a sessional basis, just as they do with non-clinical employees, such as receptionists.

Regulation of herbal remedies

Herbal remedies are regulated in three ways – as licensed herbal medicines; as unlicensed herbal medicines, or as food supplements – with different requirements for products in each category. Unlicensed preparations are thought to account for 80 per cent of all herbal sales. Licensed herbal medicines are assessed for safety, quality and efficacy in a similar way to conventional medicines (under the Medicines Act 1968, which also deals with homeopathic remedies), and have a product licence number (PL) marked on their packaging. The licence will include specific indications for use, and claims based on these can be made about licensed herbal medicines. Unlicensed herbal medicines do not have to comply with any specific safety and quality standards (under section 12 of the Medicines Act 1968). However, no written claims about their use or effectiveness are allowed on their labels. Food supplements are not subject to any rigorous safety, quality and efficacy assessments either. But they can make claims that suggest a health benefit. This all looks set to change when the new European Directives come into force (see page 41). In addition, also under Section 12 of the Medicines Act 1968, herbal medicines that are manufactured, sold or supplied by someone in a face-to-face transaction do not have to be licensed. Also, a herbalist does not have to list the ingredients in any remedy he or she prescribes; the product's safety and efficacy are the responsibility of the herbalist.

'Consent' in medical practice

Before any practitioner prescribes any medication or applies any form of lotion or substance or lays a hand on your body, it is vital that he or she ensures that you are aware of what is going to happen, what the nature of the treatment might be and what risks (such as common, mild side-effects as well as rare, severe adverse events) could arise from it; all of this should be discussed before treatment begins so that you can give your consent to the treatment.

If something happened to you which you did not expect and to which you had not agreed, there are two options open to you:

1. you can claim for damages for **failure to warn**. This will be a civil action and usually comes under negligence
2. the police/Crown Prosecution Service can bring a charge of **battery and assault**. An **assault** is committed 'when the defendant intentionally or recklessly causes his victim to apprehend the immediate infliction of unlawful force'. It is sufficient in law if the victim anticipated violence. **Battery** is committed when the defendant 'intentionally or recklessly inflicts unlawful force'. A battery may follow an assault. The slightest touching, if unlawful, may be sufficient to amount to battery. In one case (Lord Lane C.J. Faulkner *v* Talbot 1981) it was ruled that battery was 'any intentional touching of another person without the consent of that person and without lawful excuse. It need not necessarily be hostile, rude, or aggressive.'

Assault and battery are summary offences, tried in a magistrates' court with maximum penalties of six months' imprisonment or a fine, or both. Where the violent act amounts to a criminal offence, you may obtain damages through the Criminal Injuries Compensation Scheme, or alternatively pursue a claim for personal injury through the civil court. It would be advisable to contact the police, especially if you wish to bring a prosecution for criminal assault.

Anyone suffering a personal injury may bring a claim for compensation and damages against the person who caused the injury. Physical injury includes psychological damage, provided that the damage is a recognised psychological condition (the most obvious example is post-traumatic stress disorder). If you are physically injured as a result of a treatment, or feel that the practitioner breached the legal duty of care to which he or she is bound, you may have a civil claim for negligence against the practitioner under medical law.

In order to establish negligence, you have to prove that the practitioner owed you a duty of care and that he or she was in breach of that duty of care. Any practitioner who enters a therapeutic relationship with a patient, whether the medicine he or she practises is mainstream or complementary, owes that patient duty of care. You must also show that you suffered injury and that the injury was caused by the negligence of the practitioner. A practitioner must exercise a reasonable degree of skill and care.

If the practitioner conducted his or her treatment in a way that any reasonable person with those skills would have conducted it, then your case for negligence would collapse. You have to show that no professional person of ordinary skill would have done the same. A practitioner is not guilty of negligence simply because he or she did not have the highest level of skill. It is vital that, before you start on the long and expensive road of litigation, you make sure that you have a case. For that an expert is needed, who can tell you and your solicitor whether the treatment received fell below the standard of a reasonably competent practitioner. If your case is in any way weak, the defendant's expert witness will pick up on it.

Rights of access to health information
After you have an initial consultation with a solicitor, he or she will try to obtain the notes and records that the practitioner kept of your

visit. Three statutes grant specific rights of access to health information – the Data Protection Act 1998, the Access to Medical Reports Act 1988 and the Access to Health Records Act 1990. A patient has the right to obtain medical records held by 'health professionals' as defined in Section 2 of the Access to Health Records Act. This is subject to the Data Protection Act, which provides for an individual's right to see personal data. There can be no justification for a practitioner to withhold any patient's notes. Most notes are obtained under what is called 'pre-action discovery' under Section 3A of the Supreme Court Act 1981.

If the practitioner is loath to release the notes, it can take some time to get access to them. The papers will then be referred to an expert for a full report as to whether there is liability or not. An expert's report can cost anything from £300 to £1,000 depending on whether or not he or she will need to examine you. If the expert believes the case is not strong enough for a claim, it will go no further.

Product liability

The Consumer Protection Act 1987 applies to unsafe or defective products. Under the terms of the Act, a product is considered defective if 'the safety of the product is not such as persons generally are entitled to expect'. Under product liability legislation the manufacturer is liable; the shop where you bought it is liable only for own brands and when someone further up the chain cannot be identified. However, the onus is on you to show that the product is defective. The lotion that you were given by the practitioner or bought off the shelf may well have given you a rash, but if when analysed it is found to be harmless, you will have no case.

Litigation against a complementary therapist

Legal action can be a long, harrowing and expensive process. It can take two years or longer, and although your solicitor will do most of the work you will be expected to take an active interest and will have to deal with letters and attend meetings. You may have to be examined by a doctor or therapist acting either for you or for the practitioner concerned. Nevertheless, if you have the right solicitor, a strong case and the support of your family and friends, and you are fully aware of the problems that may arise, you should not be dissuaded from taking legal action.

If you fail to get better after your treatment, theoretically you have no redress under the law because you have made the decision to trust and accept the professional judgement of the therapist you have consulted. If the therapy does not work, it is up to you to go elsewhere. However, at the same time, the practitioner is contracted to give you a service. You have paid money for this, possibly over a long period of time, and it constitutes a contract. If you feel that a practitioner has not given you the agreed service, you can sue under civil law, as the practitioner has failed in his or her duty of care.

In addition, despite the fact that complementary therapists are unregulated, they have a legal duty of care towards their patients, the breach of which could give rise to an allegation of negligence. If you have suffered personal injury at the hands of a complementary practitioner, you have three years from the date of the accident or event in which to start legal action. If, however, there has been a breach of contract, whereby the service provided was defective but you did not suffer any injury, you have six years in which to sue. If the incident happened when you were a child or teenager, you have until you are 18 years old to bring an action.

On the basis of anecdotal evidence, it appears that cases of negligence against complementary practitioners are increasing, but the numbers that come to court are negligible. About 2 per cent of all claims brought against the NHS for medical negligence reach trial. The rest evaporate, either because the claimant's expert says there is no case, because the plaintiff (victim) withdraws or because there is an out-of-court settlement.

There are three reasons why people are reluctant to go to a lawyer after they have received bad treatment from a complementary practitioner. They might fear the legal costs and time involved, be ignorant of their rights or may suffer from inertia. In addition, so little has been written about what is right and what is not right in terms of treatment and how you should feel afterwards in the different spheres of complementary medicine, you may not be sure whether what happened to you is acceptable or not.

The burden of proof falls on the patient (claimant) to demonstrate that the practitioner was negligent and that this caused the damage for which you are now suing. However, there can be an imbalance between the parties in terms of their resources, extent of clinical knowledge and the difficulties they face finding reputable experts prepared to give evidence against healthcare providers. The legal standard of care is a duty to act in accordance with a practice accepted as proper by a responsible body of professional opinion. However, in the absence of nationally agreed standards and qualifications in most therapies, it may be almost impossible to define what constitutes a reasonable standard of care.

If you have had a bad experience and think you might have a good case, first you must decide whom to sue. If your GP referred you to a complementary therapist, and you subsequently fell ill or incurred personal injury, you can sue both the therapist and the doctor. You will need professional advice, though, as this is not a matter on which you should contemplate representing yourself in court (appearing as a litigant in person) or doing without legal help.

How to find a solicitor

It is best to go to a firm of solicitors that specialises in medical negligence cases and plaintiff work. The Clinical Negligence Panel★ of the Law Society, and Action for Victims of Medical Accidents (AVMA)★ each have about 100 specialists on their books. Such solicitors will know immediately to which expert the papers should be sent, what evidence to look for and how to get hold of your notes from your practitioner.

AVMA, which gives advice over the phone, produces an excellent booklet, *Medical Accidents*, containing explanations of how to complain and how to mount a legal action. The Law Society Accident Line★ has receptionists answering calls, who ask you what your case is about and give out the telephone numbers of three solicitors in your area who deal with accidents. These solicitors will then give you a free consultation of 30 minutes. Alternatively, the Law Society or your local Citizens Advice Bureau can put you in touch with an appropriate firm of solicitors, and your local library should hold a copy of the *Solicitors' Regional Directory*, which lists the names of local specialised firms.

Are you eligible for legal aid?

If you intend to make a claim for financial compensation, you will need to bring a civil action against the practitioner. The Community Legal Services (CLS)★ Fund, which replaced the civil legal aid system in 2000, is run by the Legal Services Commission (LSC)★. The LSC funds a range of legal services. If your disposable income (that is, after tax, National Insurance and providing for your family and dependants) is £611 a month or less and your capital is below £3,000 (plus dependants' allowances), you will be eligible for Legal Help, formerly known as the 'green form scheme', which will entitle you to some initial free legal advice. If you receive income support or jobseeker's allowance, you will qualify on the income criterion, but your capital will still have to be assessed. Whether or not you will qualify for a further level of aid – say, for Legal Representation, which is the new name for civil legal aid – depends on your financial circumstances and the merits of your case.

Information on the different levels of funding, the criteria for qualification, the amounts you have to pay back and a list of useful contacts is available on the LSC's website. You could also telephone the LSC's Leafletline★ to obtain relevant leaflets.

Who else might be able to help with legal fees?

You may be covered for legal expenses under your household contents insurance: around 10 per cent of people in the UK have some form of legal expenses insurance as an added extra in these policies. Many people forget that they have this cover or assume that their claim would not be covered. Most insurance companies offer legal expenses cover, some of which cover litigation concerning anything to do with your home, such as a dispute with your neighbour, and can also cover personal injury. If you are injured by a complementary or medical practitioner in any way, your insurance company may well pay your legal bill.

If you belong to a trade union it, too, may help. Many unions have arrangements with firms of solicitors and may fund an initial consultation with a solicitor or pay your legal fees up to an agreed level. But it is highly unlikely that a union will pay all your legal costs, if the problem did not directly arise from your employment.

A firm of solicitors might agree to take your case based on what is known as a 'conditional fee arrangement', that is, a 'no win, no fee' basis. Following the Courts and Legal Services Act 1990, since July 1995 solicitors have been allowed to offer conditional fee arrangements in England and Wales in the following types of cases: personal injury claims; certain bankruptcy/insolvency-related proceedings; and human rights cases (a similar system has been available in Scotland for some time). However, you must remember that although you would not have to pay your own solicitor's fees if you lost, you would still have to pay your barrister's fees, etc. and your opponent's costs (you can insure against having to pay your opponent's legal costs). You must also be aware that because the 'no win, no fee' system is risky for the lawyer, he will agree with you an 'uplift' on his bill; this means that although you will pay him nothing if you lose, if you win you will have to pay his bill in full as well as an additional amount (agreed beforehand) for winning the case, which could be anything up to 100 per cent more than the original bill. Shop around, as different lawyers will agree different 'uplift' levels. Overall, the cost of action means that a conditional fee arrangement is practically inaccessible for smaller clinical negligence claims.

Bringing a case in the small claims court

If the value of your claim is £1,000 or less for personal injury (or £5,000 for other claims), you could bring an action in the county court under the small claims procedure. A typical claim in mainstream practice might be for having sustained a minor eye injury in the course of having new contact lenses fitted at the opticians and being forced to take a week off work as a result. For such actions, you do not have to have legal representation.

To instigate such a case, you should visit your local county court, explain that you want to proceed with such a claim, and the court clerk will give you the forms to fill in and help you to do so. You will have to give a brief description of the injury and explain what financial losses you have incurred: if you were left unable to drive, you could ask for any travelling expenses incurred; you may feel you need to be compensated for the pain and suffering you have been caused; or, if you are self-employed, you may have lost work and want compensation for this.

The court would then start the process of bringing the action and serve papers on the practitioner at no expense to yourself.

District judges, who sit in small claims courts, often rely on the evidence of the claimant alone as to the level of pain or injury they have experienced.

Chapter 6

Assessing the evidence

Clearly, it is as important to have a good evidence base in the field of complementary therapies as it is in conventional medicine, particularly with the increase in use of these therapies and current moves to integrate them into the NHS. The right research can help to clearly define the role and expected outcomes of conventional therapies, and to show when and where they may be used to their best advantage, either alone or alongside another treatment. Currently, the research base in complementary medicine is small and often of poor quality, partly because some complementary therapists have been against applying the same scientific criteria to their therapies as are applied to conventional treatments, but partly because of a lack of funding and research skills in the field. However, people's attitudes are changing, both within complementary medicine and conventional medicine.

The 'gold standard' method used by scientific researchers to investigate the effectiveness of a treatment (intervention) is to conduct a 'randomised controlled trial' (RCT). However, there has been much debate about whether RCTs can be used to assess the effectiveness of complementary therapies. Randomisation is important because it creates two (or more) groups that are fully comparable. The alternative – selection – creates selection bias that leads to groups that are not comparable. In an RCT, the participants are randomly assigned to two (or more) similar groups; the experimental group(s) then receives the intervention(s) being tested and the comparison group, or control group, receives an alternative intervention, a placebo (dummy intervention) or no intervention. The researchers then measure whether the patients improve and compare the results in the different groups. Ideally, blinding is used in such trials to try and eliminate the influence of knowing what intervention the study participants are receiving. Studies can either be single-blind, when either the participants or researchers are unaware, or double-blind, when the participants and the researchers are unaware, of who is getting what intervention.

There are two main types of randomised controlled trial: explanatory trials and pragmatic trials. Explanatory trials aim to determine the exact size of the effect (efficacy) an intervention has. They are carried out in controlled conditions and rely on patients to keep closely to the design conditions of the trial. Because of the necessarily artificial setting in which such studies are carried out, their results are often not applicable to the real world. In contrast, pragmatic trials aim to determine the effectiveness of an intervention in real life, day-to-day clinical practice. They include all randomised patients in the final analysis, even if some of these patients have dropped out before the end of the trial. This is known as intention-to-treat analysis and gives a more realistic picture about the effects of the intervention.

Much of the debate about the use of RCTs to assess complementary therapies is as a result of misunderstanding about what an RCT is. Some people argue that RCTs often cannot be used because it is difficult to design suitable placebos for some complementary therapies: you can certainly give someone a dummy herbal remedy in the same way that you can give a dummy drug, but how do you give a dummy massage or acupuncture treatment? In fact, placebos are also not possible for the majority of conventional treatments; for example, most of what surgeons, nurses or physiotherapists do cannot be tested in a placebo-controlled trial. Much can be learnt from RCTs that compare different interventions with each other, rather than with a placebo treatment, and in pragmatic RCTs whole packages of treatment can be compared with each other, or with standard medical practice. Another problem that has been posed is that, in RCTs, participants within each intervention group need to receive identical treatment, which is not possible with many complementary therapies because the treatment is tailored to each patient. Again, however, pragmatic RCTs can allow for this by comparing packages of treatment rather than individual elements of a therapy. Perhaps the best proof of this is that many RCTs have been conducted in therapies as diverse as acupuncture, homeopathy, spiritual healing, yoga, fasting and reflexology.

Two other types of study are often held up as valuable measures of a treatment's effectiveness: systematic reviews and meta-analyses.

They are important because the results of RCTs very often differ, allowing proponents to select the positive ones to make their point and opponents to choose the negative studies. A systematic review is an overview of primary studies (usually controlled trials) that have used explicit and reproducible methods. Sometimes, but not always, a systematic review includes a meta-analysis of the results of the primary studies included. Done well, systematic reviews can analyse all the relevant data and can thereby offer valuable insight into the effectiveness of an intervention.

A meta-analysis is a type of trial that uses a statistical technique to summarise the overall result of two or more primary studies, typically ones that have investigated the effects of a certain intervention when used in experimental conditions. Results from the individual studies are pooled using special statistical methods to produce a single estimate of the effect of the intervention. If the primary studies and the meta-analysis are of a high standard, the conclusiveness of the results of such an analysis should be at least as high as that of the primary studies. The Cochrane Collaboration, which is an international organisation that provides systematic reviews of controlled trials looking at the effects of healthcare interventions, including those in the field of complementary medicine, has (at the time of writing) produced over 80 Cochrane reviews looking at complementary therapies and has a further 50 in the pipeline.

Funding and research skills

The main problem with research into complementary medicine has not been theoretical issues of experimental design, although many studies in the area suffer from the weakness of having very few subjects, but practical issues such as lack of funding and research skills. Very little money has been spent on complementary medicine research, and few complementary practitioners have the knowledge or experience to conduct high-quality research. Even those complementary therapists who are active in research find it difficult to compete for research funding because of a perceived or actual lack of methodological expertise and rigour. For the same reasons, research findings may not be published or accepted by conventional practitioners, which can inhibit the dissemination and implementation of the findings. The Medical Research Council*, while making it clear that it welcomes research proposals in the field of complementary medicine, states that these must compete equally with other proposals.

In its report on Complementary and Alternative Medicine, the House of Lords Select Committee on Science and Technology recommended the establishment of a central mechanism to coordinate and advise on research in the field, with funding being made available on a pump-priming basis by government, as a first step to enabling complementary medicine to build up an evidence base with the same rigour as that required of conventional medicine. The Department of Health is currently designing a national personal award scheme for complementary and alternative medicine, in order to develop the research capacity of the workforce within the field and underpin the development of its evidence base. It has stated that there needs to be created: 'an environment that supports and values the development of research skills and experience, enables access to research training opportunities and resources to undertake research activity, provides secure and attractive career pathways and encourages the development of high quality research projects.' There are also now specially designed postgraduate courses for complementary therapists to learn more about conducting research.

Do complementary therapies work?

Critics of complementary medicine often claim that there is little or no scientific evidence to support the use of any complementary therapies and that what benefits have been reported are due to the placebo effect, whereby people feel better simply because they are taking a remedy or having some other form of treatment for their condition. This is dismissive not just of complementary medicine, but also of the placebo effect, the power of which orthodox medicine is only just beginning to recognise and harness.

Research generally aims to answer questions that are much more specific than 'Does it work?' and it is often difficult to come to general conclusions on the basis of individual studies. In fact, there is an increasing amount of evidence to support the effectiveness of several complementary therapies for certain conditions. In this book, the existing evidence, and how good it is, is considered for each individual therapy in the relevant chapter.

In summary, however, while it might seem at first that it is difficult to conduct scientific trials of complementary therapies, it can and has been done. A body of evidence has been amassed to show that each of the main therapies can be effective for at least some conditions, and some techniques have been proved to be ineffective and should be avoided. That said, there has been insufficient research on complementary therapies. Many important questions remain unanswered, including those concerning the long-term effects of treatment and the issues of which therapy might be most appropriate in a given condition. Greater investment in complementary medicine research is needed in order to answer these questions.

Part II

A guide to the key therapies

Acupuncture

Acupuncture typically involves the insertion of fine needles into specific places on the body, known as acupuncture points. Acupuncture-like techniques developed independently in several communities, but in China the technique became a key part of Traditional Chinese Medicine (TCM), along with the use of herbs, diet, exercise, massage and meditation. It has been practised in China and other Eastern countries for thousands of years. The theory of acupuncture was first documented in an ancient Chinese text – the *Yellow Emperor's Classic of Internal Medicine* (the *Nei Ching*) – which is thought to have been compiled about 2,500 years ago. Legend has it that acupuncture was discovered when physicians attending battlefields saw soldiers with arrow wounds cured of old injuries or chronic ailments. The physicians took note of precisely where the wounds were and then began to experiment by sticking fishbones and flakes of flint into specific areas of the body. It is thought that missionaries and other people returning from the colonies first brought acupuncture to Europe in the seventeenth century. However, its use did not become widespread until the 1970s. Today, the theories of medicine discussed in the *Nei Ching* still play a major part in the practice of TCM-based acupuncture; but, over the last few decades, as TCM acupuncture has increased in popularity, the use of another style of acupuncture has also increased in the West – 'medical' or 'Western' acupuncture. TCM acupuncture is practised by the 2,000 or so mainly non-medically qualified members of the British Acupuncture Council* and medical acupuncture is mainly practised by 2,000 doctors and 2,000 physiotherapists. There is some overlap between the two styles.

How does acupuncture work?

TCM is a complete healing system and embraces a totally different philosophy from that of conventional medicine. It has its own theory of what causes disease, its own system of classifying disease and its own diagnostic framework. It is based on the theory that we all have Qi (pronounced 'chee'), loosely translated as 'energy' or 'life force', flowing throughout our bodies. While Qi is said to flow all over the body, it is thought to be particularly concentrated in meridians or channels, along which lie what are commonly known as the acupuncture points (see page 72), and it is these meridians that are depicted on a traditional chart of acupuncture points. In a healthy person, Qi is said to flow freely, be evenly distributed and be neither deficient nor in excess. Illness is seen as a disharmony or imbalance due to blocked Qi, or too much or too little Qi, in the whole body or part of it. Alterations in Qi can occur at physical, emotional (mental) and spiritual levels. The concept of Qi is also used to explain physical processes in the body such as breathing and digestion, as well as how the brain works in terms of feelings and thinking.

Another fundamental concept in TCM is that of Yin and Yang. These are opposite but complementary forces whose perfect balance within the body is essential for well-being. Yin denotes cold, damp, slowness and darkness, while Yang denotes heat, dryness, action and light. It is the interaction between Yin and Yang that is said to give rise to Qi. In TCM, disease is described in terms of patterns of disharmony, most commonly using imbalances in Yin and Yang (known as the Eight Principles) as a basic matrix and also looking at signs that relate to the Organs (for example, heart, lungs, kidneys, liver, spleen), the Fundamental Substances (for example, Qi, blood, spirit) and disease factors (for example, emotions, external factors such as wind or damp, constitution, etc.). Diagnosis involves assessing a patient's Qi, while treatment involves manipulating it in some way (for example, with acupuncture). The focus of TCM treatment is on stimulating the body's own healing responses to help restore its natural balance and so improving the overall well-being of the patient and, with this, other signs and symptoms, rather than the isolated treatment of specific signs and symptoms. As such it claims to be holistic, with each treatment tailored to the individual. There

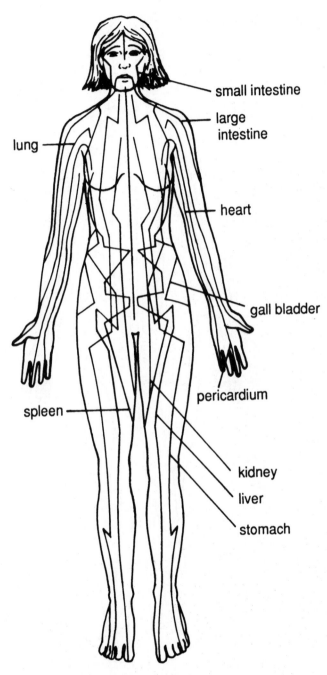

Main meridian lines on the front of the body

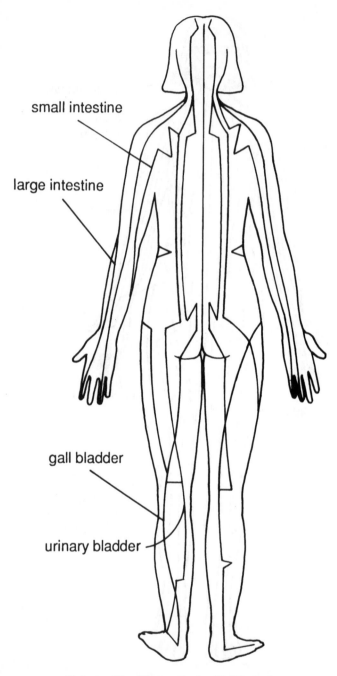

small intestine

large intestine

gall bladder

urinary bladder

Main meridian lines on the back of the body

are other approaches used by TCM acupuncturists which have also been developed as individual approaches, such as the 'Five Elements' approach, which is based on interactions and relationships between the five basic elements of the universe – fire, water, metal, wood and earth – and the 'Stems and Branches' approach, which is based on theories of Chinese astrology.

Medical (often also called 'Western', 'scientific' or 'modern') acupuncture does not always embrace the system of TCM but rather uses acupuncture techniques, and tends to apply them on the basis of a conventional medical diagnosis. Treatments mostly use a limited number of symptomatic points and focus on bringing about the relief of specific symptoms. Needles may be inserted into 'traditional' acupuncture points or into 'trigger points' unrelated to the TCM model of acupuncture. Some medical acupuncturists have dispensed with TCM theories entirely and even question whether meridians and acupuncture points exist. The favoured 'scientific' explanation of how acupuncture works is that it stimulates nerves in skin and muscle, sending impulses to nerve cells in the central nervous system to produce a variety of effects on the body's hormones, nervous system, muscle tone, circulation and immune system, and stimulating the release of substances such as natural opiates (endorphins) that can relieve pain, or anti-inflammatory substances: all these changes appear to be short-term effects. There is, however, also evidence that acupuncture can have a long-term local effect in pain reduction that builds up over weeks or months. This may be related to the responses of the autonomic nervous system near acupuncture sites as well as, perhaps, gradual changes in the content of neurotransmitters (chemicals produced in the body at nerve endings that transmit nerve signals from one nerve to another or to muscles) and hormones in the brain. Both the autonomic nervous system and the neurotransmitters and neurohormones in the brain have a profound effect on health, so this could be at least one explanation for the therapeutic effects of acupuncture. However, certain aspects of TCM acupuncture cannot be explained in conventional terms. Another, newer and as yet unconfirmed, scientific theory is that acupuncture works via connective tissue, which runs the length of the body.

Finally, auricular or ear acupuncture is widely used by TCM and medical acupuncturists alike. It is based on the theory that a map of the human body is mirrored on the ear. Ear acupuncture is used alone or in combination with full body acupuncture, and is particularly widely used for addictions. Some research suggests that needling ear points may trigger the release of neurotransmitters and hormones in the brain.

Who uses acupuncture?

All kinds of people, from the very young to the very old, use acupuncture for virtually any problem, be it physical, mental or even spiritual. Some have it to help with specific symptoms or conditions, such as insomnia, arthritis, asthma, back pain, migraines or other aches and pains; others have it as a preventive measure to keep them well and strengthen their constitution, or because they feel 'off colour' although they are not 'ill' in the conventional medical sense. It can also be used during pregnancy, but some of the points must be avoided. In China, acupuncture is also given to anaesthetise patients before planned surgery, when they usually receive a painkiller and sedative as well; this is not done in the UK, where acupuncture is increasingly used alongside conventional medicine.

Is it effective?

In a survey published in *Which?* in December 2001, 60 per cent of respondents who had had acupuncture said they had been very satisfied with the treatment, while 53 per cent said that it had greatly improved their specific health problem. Acupuncture has been assessed in more trials than almost any other complementary therapy: there have been several hundred randomised controlled trials evaluating acupuncture. The majority (but not all) of these studies show that acupuncture is significantly better than a placebo or other therapies such as drug treatment for dental pain, chronic low back pain, nausea and vomiting (after chemotherapy or surgery) and migraine. In fact, in a book published by the British Medical Association, Professor Edzard Ernst has suggested that 'consideration should be given to the need for a policy, guidelines and flexible mechanisms of making [acupuncture for these conditions] available to NHS patients'. Fairly good evidence exists to show that acupuncture is not of any benefit for stopping smoking, losing weight or for treating tinnitus (ringing in the ears).

There is also evidence, albeit less conclusive as yet, from controlled trials to suggest that acupuncture may help in other painful conditions such as period pains, neck pain, arthritis and rheumatic problems, tennis elbow, fibromyalgia, tension headache and angina, as well as for asthma, recovery from stroke, high blood pressure, urinary incontinence, infertility, morning sickness and depression. The evidence for a benefit in people with drug dependence is inconsistent. Other conditions for which there is descriptive evidence, but not enough evidence to draw any conclusions about the effectiveness of acupuncture, include irritable bowel syndrome and other digestive problems, chronic fatigue syndrome, hay fever, anxiety and stress, pre-menstrual syndrome and menopausal symptoms. This does not mean that acupuncture will not work for these conditions or others not mentioned here, just that the research has either not been done yet or it is methodologically poor.

A typical treatment

The first consultation with an acupuncturist generally takes 60–90 minutes. To start with, a TCM practitioner will ask detailed questions about the condition you have come to have treated, such as how long you have had it, what, if any, type of pain you have, and if anything makes the condition worse (for example, cold, heat, certain foods, movement, pressure). He or she will also ask about your general state of health, any other problems you have and any medicines you take, your diet and lifestyle, any likes and dislikes, your emotional state and sleeping patterns, your bowel and bladder function, and your medical and family history. A TCM acupuncturist will also usually carry out a couple of standard tests – feeling your pulses and looking at your tongue, to assess the state of your Qi. The pulses are checked on both your wrists for quality, strength and rhythm; for example, a slippery pulse is said to be due to dampness in the body. The tongue is examined to assess its colour, size and coating; for example, a red tongue with no coating is said to be due to a deficiency in Yin (the cooling element in the body). Some TCM acupuncturists also press various acupuncture points to assess which ones are tender or painful. With all this information, the acupuncturist will work out what imbalances (disharmonies) you have and what the best treatment is for you. A medical acupuncturist will spend some time taking a Western medical history and may also press points to assess which acupuncture points are tender and to look for 'trigger' points.

Once the practitioner has made a diagnosis, you may be asked to undress totally or partially, depending on what points you need needling, and to lie on a couch for the treatment. There are about 500 acupuncture points altogether, from which the acupuncturist will probably choose between two and 20 points to needle in any one treatment. Needles are usually inserted in both sides of the body, to a depth of 1–2cm, but they can go as deep as 12cm, depending on which part of the body the acupuncturist is treating and how fat or muscular you are. At a nail point, for example, the needles only go in a millimetre; in the buttocks the depth could be several centimetres. Once a needle has been inserted it is usually left in place for about 15–20 minutes. During this time, it should not hurt but some people feel a tingling or dull ache around the needle. Some TCM acupuncturists try to bring on a sensation called 'de Qi' at the point of the needle by moving (manipulating) the needle when it has been inserted. This can cause a feeling that some people find unpleasant or painful.

The acupuncturist may also supplement needling with the use of moxa, a herb (mugwort) that is burnt on or over a point or on the end of a needle to warm the point (a technique called moxibustion), or may use 'cupping' – placing cups (to create a vacuum) on the skin in strategic places. Sometimes the needles are connected via wires and electrodes to a battery-operated electrical device that vibrates the needles and produces a tingling sensation, a technique known as electroacupuncture. Sometimes points are stimulated using lasers, acupressure or tuina (both forms of massage of points; see also *Massage therapy*), instead of needles. Also, sometimes tiny 'press' needles or seeds are fixed with a plaster over ear points and left in place for 1–2 weeks. A TCM acupuncturist might also give you dietary advice, exercise suggestions or Chinese herbs to supplement your treatment. At subsequent treatment sessions, your acupuncturist will probably spend 10–15 minutes talking to you before inserting the needles, the whole session taking about 30–45 minutes.

It is not possible to say exactly how many acupuncture treatments someone will need, but a rule of thumb is the longer you have had a problem the more treatments you will need. Most people with an acute problem need to have at least three treatments at weekly intervals. Those with a chronic condition might need to go weekly for about six sessions, then fortnightly for a few sessions, then monthly and so on. Most people should notice some change after five or six treatments. Some people, particularly those with chronic conditions, consult their acupuncturist for 'top up' or ' preventive' treatments, even when they are well, for example every 3–6 months, or with the change of seasons. A first consultation with a private acupuncturist will cost you about £20–£60 depending on where the practitioner is based, while follow-up sessions are usually about £5–£15 less. Some private practitioners offer discretionary concessions.

How safe is it?

Two very large studies published in 2001 in a leading medical journal concluded that acupuncture is a relatively safe treatment in the hands of a competent practitioner. Although acupuncture is one of the most invasive of the complementary therapies, serious adverse events such as infection, punctured lung or spinal cord injury are extremely rare. Such serious events are probably almost wholly due to an inadequately trained practitioner or bad practice, for example using 'dirty' needles, or inserting them wrongly, so it is important to make sure you go to a properly trained and registered acupuncturist (see below). Also, make sure that your acupuncturist uses disposable needles, which are used only once and then destroyed, to eliminate the risk of cross infection.

Conversely, mild, short-lasting side-effects, such as a slight pricking sensation when the needle is inserted, or very slight bleeding (a drop of blood) or superficial bruising, are quite common with acupuncture, although acupuncture needle insertion does not necessarily hurt in the same way that drug injections or taking blood do, because acupuncture needles are very fine (not much thicker than a hair). Many people say they feel relaxed and even sleepy during an acupuncture treatment, while some feel energised by the treatment. Other potential, but less common, minor unwanted effects with acupuncture include fainting (rectified by immediate removal of needles), nausea/vomiting (ditto), a local allergic reaction where the needle has been inserted and temporary aggravation of pain.

There are few contra-indications to acupuncture, but some points should probably be avoided in pregnancy and electroacupuncture can interfere with cardiac pacemakers. Acupuncture is inappropriate in people with uncontrolled severe bleeding disorders. Care should also be taken to avoid certain points in patients using anticoagulant medication such as warfarin. Needles that are left in place for any length of time, such as ear press needles, are unsuitable for people who have an increased risk of infection.

Finding an acupuncturist

Most people who receive acupuncture still do so privately, but use of acupuncture within the NHS is growing faster than any other complementary therapy: about a quarter of all the acupuncture treatments reported in the *Which?* survey were on the NHS, representing more than half of all the NHS-funded complementary treatments, and at an estimated cost of nearly £26 million. A majority of pain clinics and physiotherapy departments within NHS hospitals offer acupuncture and more than 2,000 GPs and hospital doctors have trained in certain acupuncture techniques.

Acupuncture is not a statutory regulated profession at the moment, and anyone can legally call him- or herself an acupuncturist and start sticking needles into people. However, members of one of the main acupuncture organisations in the UK, the British Acupuncture Council (BAcC)*, recently voted to pursue self-regulated statutory regulation, which could result in the title of acupuncturist becoming protected in law. BAcC-registered acupuncturists may or may not be medically trained, but will have had at least two, and often three or four, years' full-time training accredited by the British Acupuncture Accreditation Board (BAAB), which was set up by the Council for Complementary and Alternative Medicine* (see Chapter 4). This training includes not only TCM theories but also conventional anatomy, physiology, pathology and diagnosis. BAcC-registered acupuncturists mainly practise TCM acupuncture. The BAcC holds a register of its members, who follow a code of ethics and practice; those practising in the UK are fully covered by medical malpractice and public/products liability, and insurance.

The two other main organisations in the UK are the British Medical Acupuncture Society (BMAS)*, whose members are doctors, and the Acupuncture Association of Chartered Physiotherapists (AACP)*, whose members are physiotherapists. These practitioners mainly use medical acupuncture, and have already worked extensively in conventional medicine. They have statutory regulation as doctors or physiotherapists. The BMAS offers two levels of training to its members. The first level is the Certificate of Basic Competence in acupuncture, which comprises four study days, 30 case histories, a safety questionnaire, observed safe needling technique and an oral assessment. Further specialist training is covered by the Diploma of Medical Acupuncture, which is accredited. To obtain this the practitioner must: have his or her Certificate of Basic Competence; be a medical doctor registered with the GMC, and so be covered by its code of ethics and practice; be a member of the BMAS; provide a log book of 100 cases (15 in detail); demonstrate at least 100 hours of training; and apply for re-accreditation every five years. The AACP has a code of practice over and above that for state-registered physiotherapists. Basic members require 80 hours of training; advanced members 200. Moreover, members of the AACP are required to keep up with a stated minimum number of training hours per year in order to remain on the register, and all AACP members have approved training in acupuncture for pain relief.

Alexander technique

The Alexander technique is more of an educational process than a therapy, in that it teaches you how to improve the way you 'use' your body in everyday life and how to change postural habits. Through this enhanced body awareness, you can move and hold your muscles in the best way possible, whatever you are doing, be it sitting, standing, running, walking or even talking. By teaching you to hold yourself more efficiently, it helps you to develop a posture that is beneficial to your health and well-being. Learning the technique involves commitment and a willingness to take responsibility for the way in which you use your body.

The technique was developed by an Australian actor, Frederick Alexander (1869–1955), when he started having problems with his voice. By carefully observing himself in a full-length mirror and experimenting with his posture, he discovered that the way he stood affected his breathing and his voice. He noticed that the muscles in his neck would tense, pulling his head back and down on top of his spine, whenever he began to recite his lines and that this directly affected his vocal cords. Over many years, he explored how he could alter his posture to best benefit his voice and his general health. Eventually, he went on to teach what he had experienced himself.

How does the Alexander technique work?

The Alexander technique is based on the principle that each of us functions as a whole. Good posture is said to be the most efficient use of the skeleton to keep the body erect and give it freedom of movement. In short, it depends on a balanced relationship between the head, neck and spine, and is a way of standing, sitting or moving that does not put excessive strain on the muscles or joints anywhere in the body. Alexander teachers believe that we need to consciously learn to prevent unwanted, unnecessary and harmful postural habits (such as over-arching of the lower back, locking at the knees, hunched and rounded shoulders or a neck that pulls too far forwards) to improve our posture. Because we have often had these habits since childhood, and have repeated them daily, they are usually unconscious. Part of the process of learning and applying the Alexander technique is to become aware of what it is that we are actually doing and be more in touch with how we move. Good posture comes from within, and cannot be forced. A spine is made up of a series of curves that form an 'S' shape and give the back strength and resilience. Our spines should not therefore be poker straight – for 'perfect' posture, the curves need to be just right.

As well as improving your posture, the Alexander technique is restful and calming and is purported to help you regain psychological and physical poise. By releasing tension and improving breathing, digestion and the circulation of blood and lymph, the technique may also help relieve health problems such as back pain, headaches, breathing problems and anxiety.

Who uses the Alexander technique?

Many people learn the Alexander technique because they have a physical problem, such as lower back pain, whiplash, chronic migraine, joint problems, a repetitive strain injury, digestive problems, or a vocal or breathing disorder. Others learn it because of stress-related conditions or an emotional problem such as anxiety, depression, poor self-esteem or an eating disorder. The technique is also taught in music and drama colleges worldwide and, due to its positive influence on coordination, is often seen as an essential element in a performer's training. Actors, musicians and singers often train in the technique to help with their breathing, voice and pre-performance nerves: in fact, several Alexander lessons have been part of a £2 million programme funded by the British Performing Arts Medicine Trust to deal with stage fright. Sportspeople learn it to give them increased awareness in their sport and pregnant women use it to help them cope with the rapid changes that pregnancy brings.

Is it effective?

In a survey published in *Which?* in December 2001, 66 per cent of respondents who had had Alexander lessons said they had been very satisfied, while 53 per cent said that it had greatly improved their specific health problem. Many people claim that the Alexander technique gives them an experience of lengthening, expansion and freedom of movement. The effectiveness of the technique has been the subject of several scientific studies. Controlled trials found that it enhanced breathing in healthy volunteers, improved how well elderly women could reach for things, and improved performance and reduced anxiety in music students. One uncontrolled trial reported that the technique reduced pain in chronic back pain sufferers and that the effects lasted for six months. In addition, a small observational study found that it reduced depression and improved performance of daily activities in patients with Parkinson's disease. The Medical Research Council★ is currently funding a large randomised controlled study comparing the Alexander technique with massage, or standard GP care for recurrent low back pain.

A typical lesson

The Alexander technique is best learnt through the guidance of a qualified teacher and is taught on a one-to-one basis. While group introductory courses are available in many areas, these are simply to introduce the ideas of the technique and cannot offer the teaching needed to effect lasting change. The objective of the technique is to learn to maintain the poise of your head and total lengthening of your spine at rest and while moving. In the first lesson, the teacher will observe you, noting how you move, sit and stand, and will also be interested in what type of work you do, such as whether it involves sitting at a computer all day or carrying heavy loads. The teacher will then give you instructions and make gentle adjustments to your body, at rest and while you are going about everyday activities, such as standing up from a chair. The adjustments do not involve any tugging, pulling or thrusting. The teacher will simply lay his or her hands on a part of your body to bring awareness to it. Likewise the instructions do not involve asking you to make strong or violent movements. For example, if you have a tendency to hunch your shoulders, the teacher will not tell you to pull them back, but will ask you to concentrate on the muscles of your shoulders and imagine them releasing down. An example of the type of verbal instructions used is: 'Let the neck be free, to let the head release forward and up, to let the back lengthen and widen'. At first, you may find that any new positions you adopt feel 'wrong'; this is because we become used to the way we hold ourselves. So, for example, if you have held your right shoulder higher than your left for the past 20 years, this will initially feel the right way to hold it and moving the shoulders to a level position will feel wrong until you get used to it.

For comfort, it is a good idea to wear loose-fitting clothes, and trousers are more appropriate than skirts. The first few lessons will probably be concentrated on helping you look at your posture and balance while standing and sitting, and on helping you to relax by lying down on a couch or on the floor, with your head on a small pile of books and your knees raised. In later lessons, which will be tailored to suit your needs, you will probably be taught ways of moving, bending and reaching. The teacher may also help you with specific movements that relate to your work or lifestyle, such as how to sit while playing a musical instrument, work at a computer, carry heavy bags, etc.

The cost of lessons varies according to where you live and the experience of the teacher. Many teachers offer reduced rates for block-bookings or special circumstances, and lack of money should never prove a barrier to learning the technique – please contact local teachers for more information on lesson fees. Because success relies on building up a rapport with your teacher, it is a good idea to arrange a trial lesson to see whether you get on with the teacher and the technique; teachers do vary in their approach, with some explaining the technique in detail and others working more in silence. Each lesson lasts for about 30–40 minutes depending on your needs and the preferences of the teacher. The Alexander technique is not difficult to learn but does take time, so an initial course of 20–30 lessons is recommended to acquire the basic skills, ideally twice a week. You will also be encouraged to practice between lessons.

How safe is it?

Because the Alexander technique is so gentle, there are no direct risks associated with it, and it is suitable for people of all ages, whatever their state of health and fitness. The main contra-indication to the technique is a lack of commitment and motivation. It is not a 'quick fix' method and ideally becomes something that is integrated into your everyday life for the rest of your life.

Finding an Alexander teacher

Most doctors consider the Alexander technique to be of benefit for people with poor posture, stress or chronic back pain, and many GPs recommend lessons to their patients. Although you are extremely unlikely to receive tuition on the NHS, most medical insurance companies will pay for lessons if they are prescribed by a consultant. The main umbrella organisation in the UK is the Society of Teachers of the Alexander Technique (STAT)*, whose members can be recognised by the initials MSTAT. The society was established in 1958 by teachers who were trained personally by Frederick Alexander. It supervises training, upholds a code of ethics and maintains a register of teachers. There are currently about 1,130 teaching members, most of whom are based in the UK. All the members have completed a three-year full-time training course and have reached a standard approved by the society; hold professional indemnity insurance cover; and observe a published code of professional conduct. Many also attend regular postgraduate and professional development courses provided by the society. About 65 Alexander teachers in the UK do not belong to STAT.

Aromatherapy

Aromatherapy is the use of essential plant oils for medicinal purposes. Humans have been utilising essential oils in fragrances, flavours and medicines for thousands of years: records of their application go back to the times of ancient Egypt, China and India. Use of essential oils decreased in Britain with the rise of medical science in the seventeenth century. Aromatherapy as we know it now owes its development and name to a French chemist called René-Maurice Gattefosse. Apparently, Gattefosse burnt his hand while working in a perfume factory in the early twentieth century and immediately poured some lavender oil on to it. He was so impressed by how quickly the burn healed, and without scarring, that he began studying the healing powers of essential plant oils. He experimented with essential oils during the First World War and later Dr Jean Valnet carried on the work. It was Marguerite Maury, a French biochemist, who extended the research and introduced modern-day aromatherapy to the UK in the 1950s. Robert Tisserand started the first aromatherapy training institute in the UK in the 1970s.

Essential oils are not actually oils, nor are they essential. They are aromatic (highly fragrant), volatile (evaporating quickly) essences (this is where 'essential' is – wrongly – derived from), which are made up of numerous different chemicals. They can be found in the flowers, leaves, seeds, roots, grasses, peels, resin or barks of a wide range of plants. The oils are present in tiny droplets in the plant and are exuded in greater concentrations at certain times of the year and day or night. They readily evaporate, and it is the vapour from an essential oil that you are inhaling when you smell the characteristic aroma of a plant. About 400 essential oils are extracted, by distillation or expression, from plants gathered all over the world. Some of the most popular oils used in aromatherapy today include chamomile, lavender, ylang ylang and tea tree. Generally, essential oils must not be put directly on to the skin and are diluted in a carrier or base vegetable oil prior to application. Aromatherapy is often used together with massage to increase the oils' effects. The oils can also be added to baths; inhaled via steaming water, a diffuser or an incense burner; or put next to the skin in a cold compress. Also, a wide range of toiletries are now available that contain essential oils and purport to have healing properties.

How does aromatherapy work?

Essential oils are said to possess therapeutic properties that can be used to improve health and prevent disease. They are believed to work at physiological, psychological and cellular levels in the body and to be relaxing or stimulating depending on the chemistry of the particular oil being used and also on any previous associations the individual has with a particular aroma. The scientific theories for how essential oils work are based partly on the fact that they are readily absorbed through the skin and partly on the way the oils stimulate the sense of smell. Research has shown that when essential oils are applied to the skin or breathed in they are absorbed into the bloodstream through the skin or lungs respectively, and metabolised in the body in a similar way to other medicinal substances. When we smell an essential oil, this triggers the limbic system, the part of the brain that controls emotions and stores and retrieves learned memories. This could, in theory, then make us feel more relaxed and happy; however, these theories have not been conclusively proven scientifically. Some essential oils have also been shown to have antimicrobial properties.

Who uses aromatherapy?

Aromatherapy is the fastest growing complementary therapy in the UK and is now one of the most popular. It is probably most often used as a treatment for stress-related problems, pain and problems with sleep, but is also used for a variety of chronic conditions such as arthritis and rheumatism, and menstrual problems. It is becoming increasingly used in the NHS, particularly by nurses who have subsequently trained in aromatherapy. Conventional medical settings where it is available in the UK include intensive care units, coronary care units, renal units, palliative care settings, hospices and geriatric units. Aromatherapy is also widely available in health and beauty clinics and gyms. It is most often used in conjunction with massage.

Aromatherapy is also related to herbal medicine by the fact that essential oils are all extracted from herbs used in herbal medicine, and some herbalists prescribe essential oils to use externally or, rarely, to take internally. However, it is important that you never take an essential oil internally unless you have been prescribed it in this way, as it could be toxic. Properly qualified and registered aromatherapists should not dispense essential oils for oral ingestion, unless they are also suitably qualified to the equivalent standard of a medical herbalist or medical doctor.

Is it effective?

In a survey published in *Which?* in December 2001, 59 per cent of respondents who had had aromatherapy said they had been very satisfied, while 43 per cent said that it had greatly improved a specific health problem. Aromatherapy is claimed to help a wide range of health problems from anxiety and insomnia to asthma and eczema, although most of the evidence is anecdotal. However, a systematic review of six randomised controlled trials of aromatherapy suggests that it has mild but short-lasting anti-anxiety effects. There is also some promising, but inconclusive, evidence that aromatherapy can help a type of baldness called alopecia areata (at least applying an oil to the scalp may help), and that it might help prevent bronchitis. Tea tree oil has been shown to help relieve acne and fungal infections. Peppermint oil is available on an NHS prescription as a conventional medicine to treat abdominal colic and bloating, particularly in irritable bowel syndrome. More research is needed to investigate the effects of aromatherapy for other conditions.

A typical treatment

At an initial aromatherapy session, the aromatherapist will probably take a detailed medical history and ask questions about your diet, lifestyle and any health problems you may have. You may also be asked about any aromas you particularly like or dislike. Based on this information, the therapist will then decide which essential oils are most appropriate for you as an individual (this may be one oil, or a blend of two or three). Aromatherapists are not, however, trained to make a medical diagnosis. The therapist will then usually blend the chosen oil(s) into a carrier oil such as almond or grapeseed oil, often at a dilution of 2 per cent, and massage this mixture in to your skin. He or she may perform a patch test on your skin first to make sure you are not sensitive to any of the oils chosen: this is particularly wise if you have sensitive skin or are prone to allergic reactions. A good aromatherapist will have a large selection of oils from which to choose. The massage techniques used are usually like those used in classical massage (see page 129). The therapist may also give you advice about what oils you could use at home, for example, in the bath or as an inhalation. A session normally lasts for 60 to 90 minutes, and costs between £20 and £40. The number of treatments will depend on what you are trying to achieve. You may just want a relaxing massage, in which case one session is enough; for a chronic condition, you will probably be recommended to have one treatment a week for a few weeks, then follow-ups after two or four weeks. Most people feel some benefit after a couple of sessions. Some people feel slightly disoriented or light-headed after an aromatherapy treatment, but most simply feel relaxed.

How safe is it?

Essential oils need to be used with care because they are very concentrated and can be toxic if used incorrectly. However, there are probably few risks associated with aromatherapy when it is practised by a responsible and properly trained therapist. Side-effects include headaches, feeling sick, and allergic reactions. A few oils, such as those from the citrus family (for example, orange, lemon, bergamot), can cause photosensitivity, where your skin burns more easily in sunlight because the oil reacts with ultraviolet light. If you have had such an oil applied to your skin, avoid direct sunlight. Essential oils should almost never be used neat on the skin (except for lavender or tea tree oils in small amounts in an emergency situation) and should only be taken internally on the advice of a fully trained medical herbalist (see pages 116–7). A few of the oils are potentially carcinogenic.

If you are pregnant or breast feeding, it is important to check with a professional therapist or your doctor or pharmacist first before using an essential oil, because there are several essential oils that should not be used during pregnancy and some that may get into breast milk. Some oils can aggravate skin conditions in susceptible people, and essential oils should be used with extreme caution, or not at all, on infectious skin conditions, varicose veins and broken skin, and by people with epilepsy, a deep vein thrombosis (blood clot in the leg) or those who have recently had surgery. Never self-treat yourself if you have any of these conditions.

Some essential oils are thought to interact with certain conventional medicines, such as antibiotics, antihistamines, sedatives and anti-epileptics, to either reduce or enhance their effects. Always check with your doctor or pharmacist before using an essential oil if you are on a medicine (either prescribed or bought 'over the counter'). Most homeopaths advise against using essential oils while taking a homeopathic remedy because the oils are thought to inactivate the remedies.

Finding an aromatherapist

Many health clubs, sports centres, beauty clinics, complementary therapy centres and health spas now offer aromatherapy massage, and aromatherapy is increasingly being used within the NHS, particularly by nurses, for example, in hospices and nursing homes. It may also be possible to find a private practitioner who will come to your home to give you a massage. Who you choose as your aromatherapist depends on what you want; if it is just a relaxing massage with nice-smelling oils, someone who has undertaken a short course may be suitable. However, if you want anything more, it is advisable to make sure that you are treated by an aromatherapist who has been trained at an accredited college and has some training in anatomy and physiology.

To find a suitably qualified aromatherapist contact the Aromatherapy Organisations Council (AOC)*, which was set up in 1991 as the regulating body for the aromatherapy profession in the UK. Today, it represents 13 professional associations, their accredited schools and the interests of about 7,000 aromatherapists, all of whom are members of and have been trained by one of the 13 professional associations. It has also set up the National Register of

Aromatherapists and is pursuing statutory regulation of title for the aromatherapy profession. AOC-recognised schools are required to accredit their courses through one of the professional associations and common accreditation procedures have been adopted. The aims of the AOC are to unify the profession by bringing together its various organisations; to establish common standards of training; to ensure that all organisations registered with the council provide appropriate standards of professional practice and conduct for their members; and to offer a mediation and arbitration service in any disputes involving aromatherapy.

The AOC's 'core curriculum', which defines the mandatory threshold training standards for members, consists of 200 class hours plus 15 case studies/50 treatment hours. This must be completed over a minimum training period of nine months. The AOC also has a 'competence framework for aromatherapy', which involves an expansion of the core curriculum along National Vocational Qualification guidelines to help training establishments develop their training programmes and to standardise their assessment procedures. There is now also a BSc degree course in aromatherapy. Most professional associations also require their members to undertake continuing professional development at the time of membership renewal.

Using essential oils at home

Essential oils are on sale in a wide range of retail outlets from chemists and health food shops to supermarkets and garden centres. Currently, bottles of essential oil do not need to carry a danger warning, and some manufacturers do not include instructions for use. Also, not all essential oils are as good quality as others, some are diluted and some are synthetic. It is important to try and check that an oil has not been diluted, which can be difficult as not all manu-facturers state whether oils are pure nor whether they are synthetic. However, reputable companies only supply pure essential oils. Oils vary enormously in price but if you find a brand of an essential oil that is much cheaper than the same oil in another brand, it may be because it is diluted or has been mixed with a synthetic fragrance. An independent self-regulating body called the Aromatherapy Trade Council (ATC)★ was set up in 1993. It represents about three-quarters of the suppliers of essential oils and aims to maintain high standards among its members to ensure quality in their products. The ATC has drawn up definitions, used by trading standards authorities, of what constitutes an essential oil (that is, an aromatic, volatile substance extracted by distillation), an 'absolute' oil (that is, a substance obtained by solvent extraction) or an aromatherapy oil (that is, an essential oil mixed with a carrier oil). However, there is still no definition of what an aromatherapy product is, and there are toiletry and skin-care products for sale that are described as 'aromatherapy' but only contain a tiny amount of essential oil. Oils that are most suitable for home use include chamomile, clary sage, geranium, lavender, rosemary, sandalwood, tea tree and ylang ylang. Essential oils need to be kept in tightly sealed containers and stored in a cool dark place. And, like medicines, they should be kept out of the reach of children.

Autogenic therapy

Autogenic therapy, also known as autogenic training, is a self-help technique based on a series of simple mental exercises involving deep relaxation and passive awareness of your body. It is used to manage stress and relieve its symptoms, by switching off the body's 'fight or flight' system and switching on its relaxation system. It can also be used to help other mental and physical disorders by provoking spontaneous processes of self-healing. It was developed in the 1920s by the German psychiatrist and neurologist Dr Johannes Schultz, who systematically investigated whether patients could achieve a relaxed state similar to that achieved with hypnosis without actually inducing a hypnotic state (see page 124) by simply directing attention to sensations of heaviness and warmth in the limbs, common experiences during hypnosis. He found that this was possible, under certain circumstances, by using passive concentration combined with simple verbal formulas that implied heaviness and warmth. In 1932, he published the first edition of *Autogenic Therapy*, which detailed the clinical application of the six 'standard autogenic formulae' that still form the core of autogenic therapy today. The first autogenic therapy courses in the UK were held in 1979.

How does autogenic therapy work?

The core of autogenic therapy is a course that teaches simple exercises in body awareness and relaxation, which are designed to switch off the stress-related 'fight or flight' system of the body and switch on the 'rest and relaxation' system. The 'fight or flight' response is an ancient physiological reaction that prepares the human body for physical exertion in response to a perceived threat or challenge, such as the sighting of a potential predator. The pupils dilate, heartbeat increases, adrenaline is secreted, the bronchi of the lungs dilate, digestion slows down and muscle strength is increased. This response was originally designed to be short-lived. However, in today's society, with its continuous stimulation and stress, many of us live in a permanent state of 'fight or flight' and this can lead to anxiety, insomnia and many other health problems, as well as reducing our everyday performance. By switching off the 'fight or flight' response, autogenic therapy can help relieve these problems.

A key component of the training is passive concentration, a state of alert but detached awareness, which enhances the state of relaxation. Regular practice allows the body and mind to re-train their responses to stress, whatever the origins. There are similarities between passive concentration, with its emphasis on the detached observer, and some systems of meditation, such as the Buddhist technique of 'mindfulness'. However, autogenic therapy is a practical tool not a belief system. The theory is that, in this state of passive awareness, natural self-regulatory mechanisms in the body are able to function at their best, leading to a rebalancing of activity between the left and right hemispheres of the brain, and good functioning of the immune system.

Regular users of autogenic therapy report less stress and anxiety, and a greater resilience to emotional and physical upsets. Sometimes they also report more awareness of feelings, memories, intuition and creativity. This expanded awareness suggests greater communication between the left and right sides of the brain. Indeed, analysis of central nervous system activity during autogenic therapy has shown an increased balancing of the two sides of the brain and other beneficial changes in brain activity. Physiological tests have shown that autogenic therapy can cause falls in blood pressure and cortisol levels, which suggests a reduction in stress.

Who uses autogenic therapy?

People of all walks of life use autogenic therapy to improve their health or to enhance their performance or creativity. The main health problems that it is used for are stress, anxiety, phobias, depression, sleep problems, chronic pain, migraine, arthritis, premenstrual syndrome, digestive problems such as colitis and irritable bowel syndrome, bladder disorders, asthma, high blood pressure and angina. It is also taught to international sportsmen and women to enhance their performance, to airline pilots and crew to combat jet lag and fatigue, and in the business environment to optimise performance and concentration and to reduce stress. The Royal London Homeopathic Hospital offers autogenic therapy to patients suffering a wide variety of illnesses, and other hospitals are following suit.

Is it effective?

There have been several controlled trials of autogenic therapy, and systematic reviews of these trials have concluded that the therapy can help in several conditions, including asthma, digestive problems, glaucoma and eczema. However, the quality of the trials included was not always assessed. Two other systematic reviews of studies, one of autogenic therapy for high blood pressure and the other of the therapy for anxiety, both found that the overall results were positive. However, the quality of the studies included was often poor.

A typical training session

Before a course of autogenic therapy, the therapist will give you a detailed assessment, in which you will be asked about your medical history and be assessed for your psychological and physical suitability. If you are learning autogenic therapy for a medical condition, or if a medical problem emerges during the assessment, then you will be carefully monitored during and after training. Unless the therapist is medically qualified, this monitoring will be done in close co-operation between the therapist and your doctor. In any case, everyone embarking on an autogenic therapy course is encouraged to inform their GP about it. Following the initial assessment, you will be taught the basic techniques of autogenic therapy on a one-to-one basis or in a small group, over 8–10 weekly sessions. Each group session lasts about 90 minutes. After this, the aim is to practise the exercises for about 10–15 minutes three times each day, and to keep a brief daily record of experiences so that the therapist can monitor your progress. You do not need to wear special clothing and will not be asked to take up any unusual postures.

Autogenic therapy is practised in a quiet, comfortable setting in three standard postures: a simple sitting posture; a reclining 'armchair' posture; and a horizontal posture. The basic exercises consist of simple formulas that are repeated silently while you focus on the different parts of the body. The formulas are designed to concentrate your attention on the sensations associated with a relaxed state. Six basic exercises, or 'standard autogenic formulae', are taught initially, which involve experiencing feelings of heaviness and warmth in the limbs that spread to the whole body, changes in heart rate and breathing, warmth in the solar plexus region and coolness in the forehead. During an autogenic therapy course, or even during a single exercise, as your conscious self moves into the role of passive observer, it relaxes its role as a censor of unconscious material so that repressed and disturbing memories and feelings, or aches and pains connected with past physical injury, may begin to surface. Your therapist will watch closely for signs of such disturbances, and teach you simple self-help techniques so that you can 'discharge' them harmlessly.

For general problems, such as insomnia or anxiety, you may experience significant improvement within a few weeks; more deep-seated problems may take longer to respond. You will practise autogenic therapy alone or in a variety of every-day situations, for example, while travelling on a bus or at work. In the last training session, the therapist will discuss additional, personal formulas and exercises that can meet your specific needs, maybe to address a physical problem, an unwanted habit such as smoking, or a psychological difficulty such as insomnia. Many people find that the basic autogenic therapy course meets their needs but some may wish to explore the deep psychotherapeutic potential of the therapy using more advanced techniques. Autogenic therapy is available free at the Royal London Homeopathic Hospital. You can be referred by your GP or a hospital doctor. Contact individual practitioners for the private costs of the therapy.

How safe is it?

Autogenic therapy is generally very safe. Some people experience unusual sensations in the body when they first practise autogenic exercises, but these are short-lived. However, the therapy is not suitable for people with severe mental problems, such as psychosis and personality disorders, as these can be triggered or made worse by the introspection required to carry out the technique. It is also unsuitable for children under five years of age and people with severe learning disabilities. If it is being used to help treat a medical condition, autogenic therapy should only be undertaken alongside conventional treatment, and the patient monitored in case the training leads to changes that require alterations in medical treatment.

Finding a practitioner

There are no official regulations or restrictions on who can practise autogenic therapy. However, the British Autogenic Society★ (originally the British Association for Autogenic Training and Therapy, which was founded in 1984) has a register of suitably trained practitioners and aims to maintain adequate professional training standards. Most practitioners have other healthcare qualifications, such as in nursing, medicine or psychotherapy. All autogenic therapy therapists are required to be experienced in using the technique themselves before they train as therapists.

Biofeedback

Biofeedback is a training technique that teaches a person to self-regulate biological functions that are not normally controlled voluntarily by the conscious mind. Its aim is to help people improve their health and well-being. This is achieved by using electronic devices to observe how certain functions, such as skin temperature, respiration, heart rate or muscle tension, change in different circumstances. Its origins go back to the late 1960s in the USA, when scientists extended psychological experiments looking at conditioned behaviour to show that animals could learn to alter normally involuntary biological responses, such as the movement of the intestines, skin temperature or heart rate. Soon, people started using the medical machinery employed by scientists and doctors to monitor these involuntary responses in themselves to see if they too could learn how to affect bodily functions. It quickly became clear that humans could learn to affect their responses relatively fast and that this could result in clear health benefits, such as muscle and total body relaxation, reduced anxiety and chronic tension headaches, improved sleep and better blood flow. Biofeedback training grew in popularity and by the 1980s, in the USA, stress management courses using the training had even been introduced into some primary schools.

How does biofeedback work?

Our bodies and minds are constantly feeding back information to and from each other, but this is normally an involuntary, or unconscious, process. Biofeedback is designed to supplement this unconscious feedback by extending control into areas of the mind and body that we are not normally able to manipulate by will alone. Simple attention to biological responses is all that is required, and not any actual conscious effort, which could hinder the process. The idea is that once you can use biofeedback to affect bodily functions, you can use it in times of stress to help relieve stress-related problems such as high blood pressure or irritable bowel syndrome or avoid the physical effects of stress or anxiety such as palpitations and breathlessness.

Biofeedback can be applied to any biological response that can be monitored. The appropriate machine is attached to the person and information is then fed to the patient via a visual or auditory signal. For example, one commonly used biofeedback device, an electromyograph (EMG), picks up electrical signals from the muscles and translates them into a detectable form, such as a flashing light or a beep, every time muscles become more tense. The aim is to try to slow down the flashing or beeping, which is an indication that the muscles are relaxing. You can then learn to associate sensations from the muscle with levels of stress and develop a new, healthy habit of keeping muscles tense only as necessary, and to repeat this response at will without being attached to a machine. Other biological functions that are commonly monitored and used in a similar way to help people learn to control their physical functioning are skin temperature, heart rate (measured by an electrocardiograph), blood pressure (measured by a sphygmomanometer), sweat gland activity (measured by galvanic skin response), respiration (measured by a stretch gauge) and brainwave activity (measured by an electroencephalograph). Sometimes biofeedback is used in conjunction with other techniques such as relaxation or meditation.

Who uses biofeedback?

Biofeedback is most commonly used to treat problems that may be helped by reducing stress and tension, such as anxiety, insomnia, epilepsy, depression, asthma, disorders that may be affected by altering biological function such as addictions, high blood pressure, irritable bowel syndrome, Raynaud's phenomenon and incontinence, and conditions that are associated with muscle tension, such as chronic pain, cerebral palsy, dysphagia (difficulty in swallowing), fibromyalgia, neck and back problems, and tension headaches. Biofeedback is used in many hospitals around the UK, with 'stress management' instruments most often found in psychology departments, and the EMG instruments in physiotherapy and occupational therapy departments. Many independent practitioners also use biofeedback equipment and techniques with their patients.

Is it effective?

Although most people initially viewed biofeedback with scepticism, research has conclusively shown that we can alter our involuntary biological responses by being 'fed back' information about what is occurring in our bodies, although the precise mechanism for this is not fully understood scientifically. Some clinical trials and many observational studies have also been carried out looking at the effectiveness of biofeedback. Systematic reviews of such research into biofeedback for tension headaches and migraine suggest that it is more effective than relaxation alone and that the combination of biofeedback and relaxation is more effective than either therapy alone. Controlled trials have shown that it can be used to relax shoulder muscles and relieve muscle tension in the lower back. Other studies have shown that people can use it to learn how to control incontinence, that it may help relieve the symptoms of premenstrual stress, Raynaud's phenomenon and constipation, and that it can help people with panic and anxiety control these states to the point that they no longer interfere with daily life. In one study, 80 per cent of individuals with high blood pressure who underwent biofeedback training reduced their prescription medications or no longer needed them at all, even after years of taking medication. More than 700 groups worldwide are using EEG biofeedback, sometimes called neurofeedback, to treat attention deficit hyperactivity disorder, with reports of a significant improvement in behaviour and a reduction in medication requirements. There are also anecdotal reports that biofeedback has helped people who have been told they will never walk or use their hands again, and research is currently looking into its effects on heart rate and some US doctors are using it to treat epilepsy.

A typical treatment

You can buy a biofeedback machine and teach yourself how to use it, but it is probably best to have some sessions with a specialist first.

During the first treatment session, which takes about an hour, the practitioner will take a standard medical history, as well as ask about lifestyle and family history, and then will probably discuss the role of stress in your problem. Electrodes or probes will then be used to attach you to the biofeedback device and signals, such as beeps, flashes or needles on a dial, will then feed back information about changes in your body. Some of the newer biofeedback devices connect to personal computers and make use of multimedia feedback including animations, games and music. You will either sit up or lie down during the session. The practitioner will show you how to use the biofeedback device and to recognise signals that suggest relaxation. For example, a state of relaxation is indicted by a slow, even heart rate, high levels of alpha waves from the brain, warm skin, lowered blood pressure and low sweat-gland activity. Most people attend weekly to have their condition monitored and repeat the biofeedback practice: it takes practice to learn the biofeedback technique and most people need between four and ten 30–45-minute sessions. You may also be encouraged to practise at home, for which you can buy your own device. However, most people can eventually self-regulate their body functions without the aid of the device. To find out how much biofeedback costs contact individual practitioners.

How safe is it?

There are no known contra-indications to biofeedback, but because it can induce changes in mental state, people with psychosis or severe personality disorders should only use it under medical super-vision. Biofeedback seems relatively safe, but there have been occa-sional reports linking it with dizziness, disorientation, acute anxiety and floating sensations. If you are on any medication that affects a body function such as an antihypertensive for high blood pressure or insulin for diabetes, it is important to tell your doctor before you have biofeedback, as it may result in a need to change the dose of your medication.

Finding a biofeedback practitioner

Originally, most biofeedback practitioners were psychotherapists or counsellors but now it is used by a wide range of healthcare profes-sionals, such as physiotherapists, social workers, stress counsellors and occupational therapists. In the UK, there are no official restrictions on who can practise biofeedback and no umbrella organisation regulating practitioners. There is an organisation based in the Netherlands, called the Biofeedback Foundation of Europe★, which runs courses and has some information about how to find a practitioner or purchase a biofeedback device.

Chiropractic

Chiropractic is a manipulation-based therapy that was developed by a Canadian healer, Daniel David Palmer, in the late nineteenth century. The story goes that he manipulated the neck of a local man and allegedly cured his deafness. However, spinal manipulation has been used as far back as 400BC and by bonesetters throughout history. Indeed, Hippocrates is reputed to have said 'Look well to the spine for the cause of disease'. Chiropractic has a lot in common with osteopathy, and the differences between the two therapies are mainly historic: chiropractic focused more on the joints of the spine and the nervous system, while osteopathy lay equal emphasis on the joints and surrounding soft tissue such as the muscles, tendons and ligaments. Also, chiropractors typically use manipulation, while osteopaths use more mobilisation techniques which are more gentle. The word 'chiropractic' derives from the Greek words *cheir*, meaning 'hands', and *praktikos*, meaning 'practice'. Today, there are about 1,800 chiropractors across the UK.

How does chiropractic work?

Chiropractic is concerned with the diagnosis, treatment and prevention of mechanical disorders of the muscles and joints, and the effects these disorders have on the function of the nervous system and general health. Chiropractors typically take the view that improving the function of the musculoskeletal system by physical means is likely to benefit people with common disabilities. They use manipulation, mainly of the spine, combined with advice about lifestyle, fitness, exercise and work, to improve joint function and mobility. Many increasingly recognise the psychological and social influences on people's quality of life and well-being, and take a holistic approach to health. Some, however, take the more fundamental view that many health problems can be traced to intrinsic dysfunctions in the spine, and seek to detect and correct them. The aim with manipulation is to free joints and release tension in surrounding muscles.

McTimoney and McTimoney-Corley chiropractic are two variations of chiropractic that use very gentle and swift techniques, that appear to the observer (and usually to the receiver) to be extremely light. The key to the success of the adjustments, however, is the speed, dexterity and accuracy with which they are delivered. McTimoney chiropractors utilise an adjustment known as the 'toggle torque recoil', which effectively frees the joint and releases tension in surrounding muscles. As the manoeuvre happens very fast, patients feel almost nothing. The practitioners of these types of chiropractic also put more emphasis on a holistic approach to health and on self-help. These types might be more suitable for babies, young children and older people.

Who uses chiropractic?

Chiropractic is mainly used to treat back and neck problems, although chiropractors sometimes treat other problems caused by the dysfunction of the spine, such as headaches, migraines, vertigo and tinnitus. Some practitioners also treat the disabilities associated with arthritic conditions, sports injuries, digestive problems such as irritable bowel syndrome, asthma and period problems.

Is it effective?

In a survey published in *Which?* in December 2001, 68 per cent of respondents who had had chiropractic said they had been very satisfied, while 69 per cent said that it had greatly improved a specific health problem. There is little scientific evidence to back up the theory that spinal dysfunction is the cause of many or all illnesses, but spinal manipulation has been shown to have several biological effects such as reducing muscle spasm and pain. Chiropractic is one of the most well-accepted complementary therapies by conventional medical practitioners. Many clinical trials and systematic reviews of chiropractic spinal manipulation have been published. A recent one, which analysed the best evidence available, suggested that spinal manipulation is effective in the short term for acute low back pain. It also found it to be effective for chronic low back pain when compared with placebo and commonly used treatments such as those used by GPs, but found that the evidence was inconclusive for mixed acute and chronic low back pain and for sciatica. Other systematic reviews of chiropractic for low back pain have arrived at more negative conclusions.

A systematic review of spinal manipulation for headaches suggested that it could be helpful but none of the studies included was of high quality, throwing considerable doubt on the results. There are fewer trials of manipulation and mobilisation techniques for neck pain and the results of these trials vary. Also, very little research has looked at the effects of chiropractic on other health problems and the quality of those that have is too poor to provide any firm conclusions. There is some evidence for a beneficial effect in the treatment of period pains (dysmenorrhoea).

McTimoney and McTimoney-Corley chiropractic have yet to be the subject of rigorous research.

A typical treatment

The first session with a chiropractor usually lasts about 30–90 minutes and subsequent sessions about 15–20 minutes. At the first session, the chiropractor will ask you about your medical history and give you a thorough physical examination: you may be asked to undress down to your underwear for this. During the physical examination, the chiropractor will assess how your spine and other joints are working and look for any muscle tension, misalignment or sign of injury, while you are sitting, standing, walking and maybe carrying out other movements. The practitioner will probably also feel your spine before, during and after movement, and may assess your muscle function, test your reflexes with a reflex hammer and measure your blood pressure. Some chiropractors also use X-rays (only if essential for the purposes of diagnosis) and other standard medical tests to help them make a diagnosis. If your chiropractor thinks you have an underlying disease that needs to be investigated further, you will be advised to see your GP.

Treatment takes place with you sitting or lying down in various positions on a specially designed couch, usually with your outer clothes removed. Sometimes a chiropractor will wait until the second session before starting treatment so that X-ray results are to hand. Chiropractors mainly use manipulation and (less often) mobilisation on the spinal column and pelvic area to realign the spine. Some manipulation techniques use short, rapid movements called high velocity thrusts to spinal joints to extend them slightly beyond their normal passive range of motion. When a manipulation is performed, you may hear an unnerving click. This is not the bones cracking, but is said to be caused by gas bubbles in the synovial fluid within the joints bursting under pressure. Immobilisation techniques may be used, which, by contrast, involve the application of force to spinal joints and surrounding tissues without any thrusting movement and within the normal passive range of movement. While chiropractors do focus on the spine, they also work on other joints.

Your chiropractor may show you exercises to do at home and suggest ways you can improve your posture; some practitioners also give nutritional advice. The number of sessions needed is highly variable and depends on your particular condition. Generally speaking, you may need 3–6 treatments for simple low back pain that you have had for a short time. For a longstanding (chronic) condition you may need up to 12 treatments. Your chiropractor may also recommend that you have follow-up treatments at regular intervals to prevent your problem coming back. Costs range from about £20 to £50 for the first consultation, depending on your location, and a little less for subsequent treatments.

How safe is it?

The most serious potential risk with manipulation, if done next to the neck, is a stroke caused by injury to one of the arteries leading to the brain. Spinal cord injury caused by compression of a nerve in the spine is another serious complication. While these events are probably extremely rare, it is not actually known how often they occur and there have been calls for research to quantify the risk. More common (occurring in up to 50 per cent of treatments) but less serious side-effects include mild pain or discomfort at the site of manipulation, mild headaches or tiredness. These are regarded as a perfectly normal reaction to the body realigning, and they usually disappear within 24 hours of the treatment. There are some conditions where forceful manipulation should not be carried out; people who have osteoporosis of the spine (i.e. many older people), a malignant or inflammatory condition of the spine, osteoarthritis of the neck or a bleeding disorder, and those on anticlotting medicines and pregnant women should avoid chiropractic. Chiropractors are trained to check patients for these and other risk factors, but osteoporosis is readily diagnosed only when it is very advanced. No definite identifiable risk factors exist to predict who will suffer a stroke after manipulation. If you have one of these conditions, other low force manipulative techniques may be suitable.

Finding a chiropractor

Chiropractic is now a statutory regulated profession, so only practitioners who are registered with the General Chiropractic Council* (GCC) are legally allowed to call themselves chiropractors. Training is predominantly via degree courses over four years. New chiropractic graduates can become registered if they have completed a course recognised by the GCC. All chiropractors are required by law to be insured. If you go to your GP with back pain, you will usually be referred to a physiotherapist, who may have a long waiting list. But there is nothing to stop a doctor referring you to a chiropractor for treatment, and this course of action is increasing, with around a fifth of chiropractors now able to see patients under the NHS. In April 1996, the Department of Health launched a pilot project among 28 GP-fundholding practices across England to test the possibility of buying in the services of osteopaths and chiropractors. In September 1996, the Royal College of General Practitioners issued guidelines to GPs for the management of back pain. These recommend manipulative treatment within the first six weeks for patients who need help with pain relief or who are failing to return to normal activities.

Most people, however, see chiropractors privately, and many health insurance companies will now pay for chiropractic treatment if you have a referral letter from your GP. If you decide to find a chiropractor by yourself, check that the practitioner is registered with the GCC to be assured that he or she has undergone the required training and is fully insured to practise.

Healing

Healing is a positive interaction between one person (the healer) and another (the patient) with the intention of the healer bringing about an improvement in the other person's health and well-being. Based on a belief in a universal healing energy, most cultures and civilisations have embraced healing, with the earliest known reference to universal healing energy dating back to India in 5000BC. There have also always been healers – Jesus being the most obvious example – in Christianity. Healing energy has also been attributed to special places such as Lourdes in France and other shrines. In the UK, healing is the most extensive therapeutic system outside mainstream medicine, and today, nearly 15,000 practitioners are registered with healing organisations, and probably as many again who work independently of such an organisation. There are several traditions of healing, such as spiritual healing, faith healing and reiki; therapeutic touch is a similar skill taught mainly to nurses. It is also claimed that healing can be practised at a distance.

How does healing work?

Healing encompasses a wide range of belief systems. Many healers believe that the beneficial health effects of healing are due to the channelling of 'universal energy' via the healer to the patient. This energy is described as coming from various sources, such as the cosmos or from a religious source, depending on the type of healing, while some healers believe that there is only one 'healing' energy and this is just given different names by different healing approaches, such as prana in yoga and Ayurvedic medicine or Qi in Traditional Chinese Medicine. In all approaches, healers believe that healing helps patients heal themselves and is holistic, affecting the body, mind and spirit.

Healing is said to penetrate the deepest levels of a person's being, where many illnesses have their origin. The theory is that symptoms start to disappear as the cause is revealed and removed. Changes in attitude and quality of life may then also follow. Apart from faith healing (see below), it is not necessary for the patient to have 'faith' for the healing to work. In fact, you can be a complete sceptic and still have other forms of healing.

In **spiritual healing**, healers focus their attention on the highest source of 'Peace' and 'Love' in the universe that they can imagine. This is called attunement to the universal source and is similar to meditation; it is a state of heightened awareness, of being totally present and at the same time having an attitude of detachment. The healers then consciously direct this experience of union with the universal source through themselves to the patient. This is called channelling. This type of healing is sometimes called 'laying on of hands', although the hands are usually held a short distance from the body. At the end of a spiritual healing session, healers will consciously break the connection they have made with their patients and resume their normal everyday conscious state of being. Spiritual healing practised when the patient is not present is called distant healing, or absent healing. It can be practised in groups or individually and may involve prayer. Radionics is one type of absent healing that believes it is possible to tap into a person's 'energy' at a distance to diagnose and treat them.

The principle behind **faith healing** is belief or faith in the intervention of a higher power to promote healing. It is often associated with prayer and the 'laying on of hands' in a religious setting.

Reiki is a system of healing that was developed in Japan and uses both the 'laying on of hands' type of healing and distant healing. It is said to have its basis in ancient Tibetan Buddhism, and was apparently rediscovered in the late nineteenth century by Dr Miao Usui, a Japanese theologian. Practitioners are initiated in reiki healing and then can draw on 'reiki energy' during a treatment, which they channel into areas of need in themselves and their patients. Reiki is claimed to work on an atomic level, causing molecules in the body to vibrate with a higher intensity and so dissolve energy blocks that are said to cause disharmony and disease in the body.

Therapeutic touch has been described as a 'modern day' type of healing. It was developed in the USA during the 1970s, then introduced to the UK in the 1980s by a nurse. It is usually practised by nurses and other health professionals. Unlike other types of healing, therapeutic touch practitioners do not see themselves as an instrument for channelling healing energy, but see healing as a mutual process of exchange of energy between the practitioner, patient and the environment. They believe that we all have unique energy fields, which interact with other people's fields and the energy around us. The aim of therapeutic touch is to rebalance any disruptions in these fields.

Who uses healing?

Healers say that healing can help with most health problems – physical pain and emotional conditions are the most commonly treated problems – and is suitable for anyone. Healing is now often available in GP surgeries, NHS hospitals and hospices, as well as in healing centres and natural health centres. Since December 1991, the Department of Health has allowed spiritual healers to practise in GP surgeries, provided the GP is clinically responsible for them. An increasing number of healers work in NHS hospitals, where healing is usually carried out at the request of the patient. Any patient in an NHS hospital can request healing as long as the doctor treating him or her is told about it.

Is it effective?

Healers and patients alike often report a successful outcome with healing, and people often report feeling relaxed and at peace after a healing session. Sometimes this outcome is obvious, such as the relief of pain, but sometimes the changes that occur take place at a more subtle level or in an unexpected way, for example, serenity in someone who is terminally ill or an ability to deal better with a chronic illness. Anecdotally, healing has been reported to help with the speed and extent of recovery from serious illness and major surgery, and from the effects of treatments such as chemotherapy and radiation therapy. However, like any other therapy, healing does not work for everybody, and occasionally people who experience benefit during the treatments relapse once the course is over.

There is no conclusive scientific evidence to support the existence of 'universal healing energy', although there have been experiments showing that healing can affect isolated cells and tissues and others that have shown that healing can cause plants to grow faster. Also, there are studies showing that if a healer simply goes through the motions of healing but has his or her mind on something else at the time, the healing is not 'successful'. Many trials have investigated healing in the clinical situation but the results are highly conflicting. Two systematic reviews of healing, one of which included 23 randomised placebo-controlled trials, the other 22, found that about half of the trials had positive results, suggesting that healing is effective. However, the trials were generally of poor quality, so the results cannot be relied on. Little research has been done to follow up the effects of healing in the long term. In a survey published in *Which?* in December 2001, 67 per cent of respondents who had had reiki said they had been very satisfied with their treatment, but very little research into the effectiveness of reiki has been carried out.

A typical treatment

At your first session of healing, which could last 15–60 minutes, depending on the type of healing, the healer will usually discuss why you have come and what your health problems are to gain some understanding of them. A reputable healer should also ask you if you have seen a doctor and, if not, recommend that you do. Healers do not make a medical diagnosis, although they may use their hands to 'scan your energy field' for variations such as heaviness, holes, vibrations, blockages or changes in temperature. Some healers claim to be able to see a person's aura (see Glossary) surrounding the body and can make a diagnosis from it. For the treatment, you will then be asked to lie or sit down, close your eyes and relax, and the healer will then use his or her hands to channel universal healing energy through his or her body and into yours or, in the case of therapeutic touch, to start the process of energy exchange. In some forms of healing (for example, spiritual healing, therapeutic touch) the hands are usually held just above your body, in others they are usually placed lightly on the body, for example in reiki on 12 specific parts of your body for about five minutes each. With distant healing, the healing is normally carried out at a prearranged time and the healer(s) then visualise the transfer of healing energy from themselves to the patient at this time.

A healer should be sensitive to your modesty at all times. Your healer should check if you do not wish to be touched at all, and should adjust his or her technique accordingly. Some people report sensations of heat or tingling in areas under the hands of the healer, and healers themselves often describe feeling hot or tingly as they channel the healing energy. In healing (except faith healing), nothing special is asked of you except perhaps openness to anything that happens and a degree of trust in the healer. An awareness of the need for change and the motivation to do so can also be helpful.

Usually several treatments are needed in one course, but you should start to feel some benefit after three treatments. Some healers practise in their spare time and so make no charge for their services, although they would welcome some contribution to their expenses. However, a growing number of healers work professionally and charge accordingly. A session with a healer can cost between nothing and £60; the average is £20–£25. Ask beforehand what the fee is and avoid healers who charge excessively.

How safe is it?

Generally, healing is very safe. There are rare occasions when the patient may 'feel worse' before improving, but this is thought to be an important part of the healing process, signalling a release of stress that may have gone unrecognised. Healing should be used with caution in people with psychiatric illness. An indirect risk with healing might be that it could build up false hopes and divert someone away from conventional treatment. For example, some healers believe that they can put cancer into remission, although no reputable healer would say that to a patient and, in fact, it would be illegal to do so. A healer will generally advise you to remain in touch with your doctor.

Finding a healer

There is no mandatory training for healers in the UK, though there is some voluntary self-regulation. Healing first became organised in the UK in 1955 with the founding of the National Federation of Spiritual Healers (NFSH)⋆ by the best known of British spiritual healers, Harry Edwards. The aims of the federation at the time were 'the promotion and encouragement of the study and practice of the art and science of . . . all forms of healing of body, mind or spirit by means of prayer, meditation, laying-on of hands, manipulation, etc., whether or not in the actual presence of the patient'. Today, the NFSH is the largest single healing body, with over 5,000 members. The Confederation of Healing Organisations (CHO)* is an umbrella body made up of 14 healing organisations which requires that its members have a minimum of two years' training. It also has a strict code of ethics and forbids its members to promise a miraculous cure, striking anyone who does off their membership. All members of the CHO have professional indemnity and public liability insurance. Few healers are medically qualified, but the Doctor-Healer Network* has 150 members of whom a third are doctors with an interest in healing. It is worth contacting the CHO or the NFSH for help and advice in finding a healer. It is also important to remember that a reputable healer will not make a diagnosis, claim to be able to cure you, or attempt to alter any medication you are taking without contacting your doctor. Be wary of charismatic evangelist healers, particularly if they have a mass following. Many have enriched themselves from the donations of people desperate for a cure. Many cases have been documented of people who have died as a result of abandoning conventional treatment and following treatment by a healer.

Herbal medicine

Herbal medicine is the treatment of disease using the healing properties of plants. Herbs have probably been used as medicines since human beings first walked on the Earth; even today, most people in the world still use herbal remedies rather than pharmaceutical medicines to treat themselves when they are ill, most often simply because they cannot afford modern drugs. However, people living in wealthy industrialised parts of the world are increasingly interested in herbal medicine because they consider it to be safer than drugs. Also, a considerable proportion of modern drugs are derived from plants, the best known probably being the painkiller aspirin, which originally came from the bark of the willow tree, the anti-malarial drug quinine from cinchona bark, the heart drug digoxin from foxgloves and the painkiller morphine from poppies. Pharmaceutical companies still screen new kinds of plant material for active ingredients.

In England, herbal medicine was established formally by an Act of Parliament during the reign of Henry VIII, and it is the only country in Europe in which herbalists can practise freely. The best-known work on herbalism is Nicholas Culpeper's *English Physician and Complete Herbal*, published in 1653. Despite the fact that over the centuries herbalism was often criticised by the Catholic Church and fell out of favour as medicine became more scientific, interest in it was rekindled in the 1970s, encouraged by the World Health Organisation (WHO). Today in the UK, herbal medicines are prescribed by various complementary therapists. Western herbalists, sometimes called medical herbalists, use remedies derived solely from plant sources. The plants are usually indigenous to Europe but, increasingly, plants from around the world are included.

Chinese herbalists mainly use remedies from the Far East and include ingredients derived from plant, animal and mineral sources, while Ayurvedic practitioners mainly use remedies from the Indian subcontinent, and these comprise ingredients from plant and mineral sources.

How does herbal medicine work?

Western herbalism is based on the holistic principles of treating the mind, body and spirit, and tailors treatment to the individual. It is also based on a belief that the body can be stimulated with herbs to heal itself, and is not just aimed at relieving symptoms. However, like conventional medicine, it is physiological in its approach, with different herbs being used for their effects on certain body systems; for example, a herb might be used to help the kidneys excrete waste better or to help the liver detoxify the body. Modern Western herbalists usually use similar principles to conventional medicine to make a diagnosis but, unlike conventional drugs that usually contain one active ingredient, the whole herb is used in the belief that its constituents act synergistically to increase its beneficial effects as well as reducing side-effects. Often, several herbs are used together in the belief that their combined effects are better than the sum of their individual effects. Each herb might comprise all of a plant, part of a plant, such as the leaf, flower, root or bark, or an extract of one of these.

Ayurvedic medicine is the traditional medicine of India and dates back to about 3000BC. The word 'ayurveda' comes from two Sanskrit words – *ayus*, or 'life', and *veda*, meaning 'knowledge' or 'science'. Rather than alleviating or curing illness, Ayurveda is designed to achieve good health. It covers all aspects of health and disease, and it too takes into account physical, emotional and spiritual well-being. It is concerned with the state of three vital energies or doshas. These are vata, which is made up of the elements air and ether; pitta, which is fire and water; and kapha, which is water and earth. The character of an individual depends on his or her dominant dosha. For instance, a person whose dosha is predominantly vata is likely to be creative, active, alert and restless, and will tend to move and speak quickly, but also tire quickly. When you visit an Ayurvedic practitioner, he or she will determine your dominant dosha and whether an imbalance of the doshas is present. Taste is an important aspect of treatment in Ayurveda; for example, bitter tastes are said to reduce kapha, so the herbs recommended may favour these tastes over sweet, salty or sour flavours in someone who is kapha. Herbal medicine forms just one part of the Ayurvedic system and is used, along with panchakarma (a type of detoxification therapy), yoga, massage, diet and meditation, to balance the doshas and increase prana, or life energy. Gotu kola is probably one of the most well-known Ayurvedic herbs used in the West. It is a nerve tonic and is said to help induce mental calm and clarity, and increase intelligence, memory and longevity.

Chinese herbal medicine works on the same principles as acupuncture and herbs are used, for example, to boost or disperse energy (Qi), to tonify Yin or Yang, or to cleanse, boost or disperse blood. The ingredients of a Chinese herbal remedy are said to have one of five flavours (pungent, sour, sweet, bitter or salty), five Qi attributes (hot, cold, warm, cool or neutral) and four 'directions' (ascending, floating, descending or sinking). The combination of these properties gives a herb its particular attribute or 'inclination'. One of the most well-known Chinese herbs is ginseng (Panax ginseng). The Chinese have used the root of ginseng as a tonic for over 5,000 years and its use has been widespread in the West for about 2,000 years. It is very popular with elderly Chinese people to boost energy and as a remedy for chronic lung problems. However, scientific evidence for its benefits is limited and it should not be taken in high doses: if you take it regularly, have a short break every couple of months and limit the amount of caffeine and other stimulant herbs you consume at the same time.

Who uses herbalism?

Traditionally, people have self-treated minor illnesses with herbs from time immemorial, while specially trained herbalists or healers have been used to treat more serious illnesses. This is still the case today in most parts of the world. A wide range of herbal products is for sale in health food shops, pharmacies and even supermarkets, for problems ranging from mild depression to colds and flu; however, for anything but a self-limiting minor complaint it is important to consult a qualified herbalist (see below). Qualified herbalists treat a wide range of conditions: in fact, herbalists of all backgrounds consider that herbal medicine can be used for almost anything. It is said to be particularly good for skin complaints such as eczema and psoriasis, menstrual disorders, stress-related conditions, digestive disorders such as irritable bowel syndrome and stomach ulcers, joint problems such as arthritis, high blood pressure, respiratory infections, sore throats and colds.

Is it effective?

In a survey published in *Which?* in December 2001, 45 per cent of respondents who had had Western herbal medicine said they had been very satisfied, as did 56 per cent of those who had received Chinese herbal medicine, while 46 per cent said that Western herbal medicine had greatly improved a specific health problem and 56 per cent said that Chinese herbal medicine had done so. Herbs and herbal extracts contain whole plants or parts of plants and these are known to contain active substances, or constituents. Studies on animals have clearly shown that plant medicines do have wide-ranging pharmacological effects in the body that could, for example, involve an action on certain cells or on an enzyme or hormone. However, it is often not possible to tell which constituents are active. Many clinical trials have been conducted looking at the effects in people of specific herbal remedies for a whole range of diseases, and there is now good clinical evidence for the effectiveness of several single herb preparations for certain diseases. There have been very few good trials of Chinese herbal medicine or Ayurvedic medicine.

Some herbs have been shown to be as effective as conventional drug treatment in randomised controlled trials and systematic reviews of such trials. For example, **St John's wort** has been shown to be as effective as the antidepressant fluoxetine (Prozac) for the treatment of mild to moderate depression (more recent studies suggest it is not effective for more severe forms of depression), **saw palmetto** has been shown to be as effective as conventional drugs for benign prostatic hyperplasia, and **Gingko biloba** has been shown to delay decline in Alzheimer's disease to the same degree as acetyl cholinesterase inhibitor drugs such as donepezil. The value of **hawthorn** for mild heart failure is fairly well established and evidence suggests that its effects might be similar to that of conventional drugs.

There is also good clinical trial evidence for several other herbal remedies, including a beneficial effect with **yohimbine** for impotence (erectile dysfunction), and with **African plum** for benign prostatic hyperplasia. **Garlic** slightly lowers blood cholesterol levels, so may help to lower your risk of heart disease. **Horse chestnut** is effective for the treatment of cardiovascular insufficiency and **gingko** seems to be mildly effective for peripheral arterial disease. **Black cohosh** and **chaste tree** have both been shown to help with menopausal symptoms, and studies have confirmed the benefits of **devil's claw** for joint and back pain, **willow bark** for osteoarthritis, **feverfew** for migraines, **senna** for constipation. The evidence for **cranberry** in the prevention of cystitis is marginally in favour of its efficacy, and that for **echinacea** for the prevention and treatment of the common cold is encouraging. **Ginger** seems to be effective for nausea and vomiting and also for joint pain. The evidence for **tea tree oil** in the treatment of acne and fungal infections such as athlete's foot, and for **valerian** in the treatment of insomnia. There are also some supplements, which are not strictly classified as herbs, for which good scientific evidence exists, including chondroitin and glucosamine, both of which help reduce symptoms of osteoarthritis. Many more herbal remedies are widely used and because they are not mentioned here does not mean that they are not beneficial. However, there is a lack of good scientific evidence for the effectiveness (or not) of other remedies at present.

A typical treatment

A first consultation with a herbalist, from whatever background, generally takes from 1–2 hours (and about 30–45 minutes thereafter), during which time the practitioner will ask detailed questions about your general state of health, lifestyle, emotional state, medical and family history, and likes and dislikes. Western herbalists (and many Chinese and Ayurvedic practitioners) are trained in conventional medical diagnosis, so will examine you in much the same way as a conventionally trained doctor might. Ayurvedic and Chinese practitioners will take your pulses the Ayurvedic or Chinese way and will examine your tongue and, in the case of Ayurveda, eyes and nails. They will also look at your build and features, and gauge your mood. Using this information, the herbalist will then make a diagnosis, depending on which type of herbal medicine he or she has been trained in, as outlined above.

Herbal preparations prescribed by qualified herbalists, be they Western-, Chinese- or Ayurvedic-based, usually contain several herbs and are tailored to the individual patient's needs. Depending on your condition and its severity, you may initially need to see your herbalist once every week or two, and then less frequently as you get better. Often, you will need to take a herbal preparation for two or three months before noticing any difference in your condition. The preparations come in a wide range of formulations such as syrups, tinctures, lotions, inhalations, gargles and washes. Chinese herbalists often prescribe dried herbs or powders, with instructions for use: this usually involves preparing a tang, a soup made from boiling and reboiling the herbs. A mug of this 'soup' is then taken two or three times a day, usually before a meal. The brew is likely to taste unpleasant, but usually not unbearably so. Chinese herbalists also often prescribe herbal pills.

While professional herbalists often make up the herbal preparations themselves, people treating themselves rarely make up their own remedy, as many ready-made herbal products, such as tablets, capsules, ointments and creams, are available over the counter from a health food shop or pharmacy. Some herbalists also give advice on lifestyle factors such as diet and exercise. Chinese herbalists are often qualified acupuncturists too. Ayurvedic physicians always advise on diet and lifestyle changes, and yoga and meditation are part of the treatment. The first session with a herbalist will cost about £30, then £20–£25 for subsequent sessions. The cost of the herbal remedies is extra and can vary from about £10 to £50 a month.

How safe is it?

Just because a herbal medicine is derived from natural sources does not necessarily mean it is safe. Like conventional medicines, herbs can have side-effects, can interact with other herbs and conventional medicines, and should be used with caution or not at all in certain people. Every herb will have a different safety profile. Recently, there has been much publicity in the UK and around the world about serious side-effects with certain herbs, particularly Chinese preparations. In 2001 the Medicines Control Agency's (MCA)★ advisory body, the Committee on Safety of Medicines, advised the British government that it was 'unable to give the public any general assurances as to the safety of Traditional Chinese Medicines on the UK market'. The Chinese herbal medicine aristolochia was banned in the UK in 2000 because of reports that it had caused kidney failure and cancer. A possible link has also been identified between Chinese herbal medicine (for skin disorders) and liver problems, and two patients have died as a result of developing liver failure. No single toxic herb has been identified in the cases investigated and the responses are thought to have been idiosyncratic – in other words, the patients had an adverse reaction to a substance that is normally tolerated well by most people.

There have also been numerous reports of contamination with heavy metals and adulteration with conventional medicines such as corticosteroids in some herbal products, although this has mostly been with herbs imported from China and the Far East. At the time of going to press the anti-anxiety herb kava kava was also under investigation because cases of liver damage have been linked with its use. In addition, there are issues relating to possible interactions between herbal medicines and conventional medicines; for example, St John's wort interacts with several drugs such as oral contraceptives, and gingko interacts with the anticoagulant drugs like warfarin.

Currently, under section 12 of the Medicines Act 1968, herbal medicines do not have to be licensed, as long as no claim is made about them. Also, a herbalist does not legally have to list the ingredients in any remedy he or she prescribes: the product's safety and efficacy are his personal responsibility. The MCA regulates medicinal products for human use in the UK. About 500 herbal products are licensed as medicines and, as such, have been tested for safety and quality. However, an estimated eight out of ten herbal products are unlicensed and go through no quality control. There are a few herbs that are only allowed if they are prescribed by a doctor, and some that are banned completely in the UK. A new Directive on traditional herbal medicinal products is currently undergoing approval in Europe that should make herbal medicines safer (see page 41). Under this Directive all herbs will need to be licensed and to obtain a licence the manufacturers will have to comply with safety and quality requirements. However, the herbal manufacturers will not have to supply effectiveness trial data but will have to prove that the herbal product has been used for some time, probably at least 30 years in the European Union (up to 15 years of use outside the EU can be counted towards the 30-year period). The Directive will cover medicines that are suitable for minor medical indications and used without the intervention of a medical practitioner. The product labelling will need to give systematic information about the safe use of the product and make clear that the indications are based on tradition rather than proof of efficacy.

Using herbal medicines safely

It is vital that you tell your GP or pharmacist about any herbal medicines you are taking and it is also important to inform your herbalist of any conventional medicines (prescribed or purchased over the counter) that you are taking or if you have any medical conditions. Generally, herbal remedies should be avoided if you are pregnant or breast feeding. If you do want to take a remedy during pregnancy or while you are breast feeding, ask your GP, pharmacist or a qualified herbalist whether it is safe to do so first. If you suffer any unwanted effects while taking a herbal medicine stop taking the herbs immediately and contact the herbalist again at once, or tell your GP or pharmacist about it. If any medicinal product, whether licensed or not, has adverse side-effects, it should be reported to the Medicines Control Agency; if a particular herb is deemed to be unsafe it can be banned, as was the case with aristolochia. Only buy a herbal remedy if the package states clearly which herbs it contains, and do not collect herbs in the wild unless you know what you are looking for because it is not easy to tell a poisonous plant from a non-poisonous one. Never self-treat yourself with herbal remedies if you have a serious illness, as over-the-counter remedies are not meant for serious disorders such as diabetes, epilepsy or high blood pressure. It is vital that you do not exceed the stated dose of a herbal remedy, as herbs can have serious side-effects if taken in large doses: make sure you are absolutely clear about how you should take any remedy prescribed for you. It is also important that you do not take herbal remedies for prolonged periods, as it is not known whether it is safe to take remedies over a number of years.

Finding a herbalist

In the UK, anyone can set themselves up as a herbalist but, although most herbalists are not medically trained, the majority undergo extensive training, whether they are Western based, or Chinese or Ayurvedic practitioners. It is unlikely that you would be referred to a herbalist by your GP, although this is possible in a few areas in the UK. There are also some GPs who recommend herbs to treat minor, self-limiting conditions and a few who have some training in herbal medicine. To choose a qualified Western herbalist, contact the National Institute of Medical Herbalists (NIMH)★. Members must complete the equivalent of four years' full-time training, with at least 500 hours of supervised clinical practice, and some train to degree level. Members of the NIMH are fully insured and have to abide by specific codes and ethics. Courses in herbal medicine for doctors range from two-day introductions to two-year programmes leading to a diploma in herbal medicine. There are about 40 qualified Ayurvedic practitioners in the UK: the British Ayurvedic Medical Council★ and the Ayurvedic Medical Association UK★ hold a list of qualified practitioners. Three sorts of Chinese herbalists practise in the UK – those who have had the full training, available only in China; those who have received a limited training in China and/or the UK; and those who have had little or no training. There is no easy way of telling who is a good Chinese herbalist and who is not. Unless you have some knowledge of Chinese medicine, it is almost impossible to know whether a particular school or college of medicine in Beijing or Shanghai is reputable. The only way to be really sure of a practitioner's qualifications is to choose someone from the Register of Chinese Herbal Medicine (RCHM)★, whose members must have a minimum of five years' training, including three years in Western medicine. They also adhere to a code of practice and ethics. However, only about half of the practising Chinese herbalists in the UK are on the register, and very few of the most highly trained herbalists from China belong to it. The European Herbal Practitioners Association★ (EHPA) is an umbrella organisation for herbalists from both the West and the East, and is working towards statutory self-regulation for herbal practitioners in the UK. The Ayurvedic Medical Association UK is also taking part in this process with the EHPA.

Homeopathy

Homeopathy is a complete therapy in its own right, with a different concept of disease and a different approach to the patient than conventional medicine. Illnesses are treated with very dilute preparations, called remedies, that are made from plant, mineral, metal or animal sources. The word homeopathy is a combination of two Greek words – *homeo*, which means 'similar', and *pathos*, which means 'suffering'. Homeopathy was developed by a German doctor called Samuel Hahnemann in the eighteenth century. Hahnemann was disillusioned with the medical therapies and theories of his day, many of which were of dubious benefit, such as bloodletting and purging, or highly poisonous, such as arsenic and mercury. When he discovered that small amounts of cinchona bark, the treatment for malaria, caused malaria-like fevers when he took it while healthy, he went on to test other substances on healthy friends and family members, carefully recording the sort of symptoms they caused and, so he thought, could therefore cure. These experiments were called 'provings' and led Hahnemann to observe and describe the basic principles of homeopathy (see below).

How does homeopathy work?

It is not known 'scientifically' how homeopathy works, but homeopaths believe that the remedies stimulate the body's own healing powers, known as the 'vital force'. Homeopathy is holistic and emphasises the importance of treating the whole person – mind, body and spirit – and not just the localised symptoms of the illness. There are three basic principles of homeopathy. The first, 'the law of similars' or 'like cures like', means that the symptoms of a particular illness are identical to the symptoms experienced by a healthy individual who has been given a poison, which could be given in homeopathic doses to treat the illness. For example, the poisonous plant deadly nightshade, or *Belladonna*, causes a throbbing headache, high temperature and bright red face. So, the homeopathic remedy *Belladonna* is given to people who are feverish and have a sudden throbbing headache. Following this line of thinking, *Urtica urens*, the nettle, may be used for first-degree burns, and *Apis mellifica*, made from bee venom, for hot, red, watery, stinging swellings.

The second principle is known as the 'minimum effective dose'. This arose from Hahnemann's desire to minimise the harmful effects of the drugs being used at the time and means that the lowest dose possible should be used in order to stimulate the body's own healing responses without causing side-effects.

The third principle is known as 'the principle of potentisation'. Hahnemann developed a way of making very dilute preparations from the substances he proved. First, he made a 'mother tincture' of a substance by soaking it in alcohol for several weeks and straining off the resulting liquid. Then he used some of this mother tincture to make the final remedy by repeatedly diluting and 'succussing' (vigorously shaking) it in water over and over again. The same basic process is still used today to make homeopathic remedies. A finished homeopathic remedy probably does not contain even one molecule of the original substance in it, which you would expect would render the remedy inactive. However, homeopaths claim that the more a substance is diluted and succussed, the more effective is the resultant remedy. The theory is that the vigorous shaking actually transfers energy into the water and imprints a memory of the starting material on to it although this has yet to be confirmed by research. It is this manufacturing process of dilution and succussion that homeopaths call 'potentisation'.

Remedies can come in different potencies depending on the number of times they are diluted, with the lower potencies having less powerful and shorter-lasting effects. Two main scales are used to express the strength of the remedies – the decimal and the centesimal. The gradation in the former is, as the name suggests, in tens, so a 1X dilution is a 1:10 dilution of the original mixture; a 2X dilution a 1:100 dilution. In the latter scale, the steps go up in hundreds. A 1C dilution is therefore a 1:100 dilution and a 2C dilution a 1:10,000 dilution. For mild, self-limiting complaints, most homeopaths would recommend the 'sixth potency', i.e. a 6C dilution. More severe conditions would warrant a higher potency, such as 30C or even 200C.

Who uses homeopathy?

The sale of homeopathic medicines in pharmacies is increasing by 15–20 per cent a year, with many people self-treating minor ailments such as colds and headaches with low-potency homeopathic remedies: it has been estimated that there are around 40,000 users of homeo-pathic remedies in England every year. More and more doctors are also choosing homeopathy for their patients. Referrals to the NHS homeo-pathic hospitals continue to rise, with an increase of 31 per cent in referrals to the Royal London Homeopathic Hospital in 1997 alone.

Homeopathy has been available within the NHS since the Health Service first began in 1948. There are currently five NHS homeopathic hospitals and many community-based and inde-pendent clinics where qualified medical homeopathic doctors work. Patients can be referred to these clinics and hospitals by their GPs, and the British Medical Association (BMA)★ has confirmed in its guidance to GPs that they have a duty to refer patients for homeo-pathic treatments within the NHS. This includes referrals to NHS homeopathic clinics, if the GP thinks that homeopathic treatment is clinically indicated for a particular patient.

Because homeopathy is claimed to be holistic, it is used to treat almost any disorder. The exceptions are mechanical problems such as a back problem or severe physical injury, or serious, acute or life-threatening events such as a heart attack, stroke, diabetic coma, epileptic seizure or asthma attack, and even then it could be used alongside conventional treatment. It is most commonly used to treat chronic or relapsing conditions, such as eczema and other skin problems, asthma, allergies, rheumatoid arthritis, menstrual and menopausal problems, pregnancy problems such as morning sickness, and mental disorders such as anxiety and shock. Homeopathy is also a very popular way of treating children.

Is it effective?

In a survey published in *Which?* in December 2001, 62 per cent of respondents who had had homeopathy said they had been very satisfied, while 48 per cent said that it had greatly improved a specific health problem. Despite the wide range of conditions that homeopathy is used for, it should not be considered as a 'cure all'. A growing number of double-blind randomised controlled trials have shown significant benefits with homeopathic treatment compared to placebo (dummy treatment). Studies combining the results of these clinical trials suggest that it is more than twice as effective as placebo; however, overall, it is not possible to reliably say which disorders are best treated with homeopathy, except perhaps hay fever. More research is needed before it is possible to say what specific conditions homeopathic remedies can definitely help. Also, there is little evidence available for or against using homeopathy in 'real world' situations, such as for complicated or chronic problems. It is relatively easy to conduct a trial investigating how to treat acute symptoms with a single homeopathic remedy but this does not reflect real clinical practice. Classically, homeopaths give different remedies for different individuals depending on their symptom picture. More complex trials are needed to test this practice and few have been carried out.

A typical treatment

Many homeopaths practise what is called classical homeopathy, that is, they claim to treat each patient as an individual and attempt to identify the ideal remedy for that person's general make-up or constitution. In this type of homeopathy, diseases are not diagnosed in the same way as those diagnosed by conventional doctors, although the homeopath will want to know the conventional diagnosis too. The remedy selected is based only partly on your symptoms and also takes into account your constitutional characteristics and emotional responses, and in a way the remedy selected is the diagnosis too. To do this, a classical homeopath needs to take a very detailed case history and the initial consultation can take 1–2 hours, during which time the practitioner will ask you questions about your general state of health, lifestyle, emotional state, medical and family history, and likes and dislikes. Some classical homeopaths practise complex homeopathy and prescribe a combination of remedies, rather than just one. Further consultations will usually take no more than an hour, as the homeopath will already have your background information, and generally take place 2–6 weeks after the initial remedy has been given. There are also homeopaths who prescribe on the basis of a conventional medical diagnosis or symptoms only. These tend to be conventionally trained doctors.

In an acute situation, a homeopathic remedy may need to be taken up to six times a day for a day or two, while chronic conditions may need to be treated for many months and several consultations with a homeopath may be necessary, with more than one remedy being taken. Classical homeopaths subscribe to what they call the 'Rule of 12', that one month's treatment is needed for every year the person has had the illness: in other words, the rate of the response is proportional to the duration of the disease. Most homeopaths work in the private sector and charge between about £25 and £75 for the initial consultation and a little less for follow-up sessions. Homeopathy on the NHS, however, is free at the point of care.

Homeopathic remedies are available as tinctures, lactose-based tablets, pills, granules and powders to be taken by mouth, and some also come as creams or ointments to be applied directly to the skin. Ideally, homeopathic remedies by mouth should be taken at least 30 minutes after a meal and no food or drink should be consumed for at least 10 minutes afterwards. Some homeopaths warn against using any strong tasting or smelling substances such as toothpaste, peppermint, alcohol, spicy foods or essential oils because they believe these to cancel out the effects of a remedy. Remedies should always be stored in a cool, dry, dark place, away from strong smells. Some homeopaths also use tissue salts, which are a type of homeopathic remedy made from minerals such as quartz. They are mainly used for minor ailments like coughs, colds and sore throats, hay fever, indigestion, non-serious skin conditions, headaches, stress and muscle pains. Tissue salts can also be bought and used for self-treatment.

How safe is it?

Homeopathy is considered to be extremely safe, probably because the active ingredients of homeopathic remedies are present in such low concentrations. They can be safely given during pregnancy and to the tiniest baby. However, in about 20 per cent of people, after a remedy has been taken symptoms get worse for a short period of time before getting better. This is known as a 'healing' reaction, is usually mild and short-lived, and is thought by many homeopaths to be a necessary part of the healing process. The theory behind this is that diseases get better from the inside out and from top to bottom. So, a deep-seated cure will start in the upper body and proceed downwards (for example, a rash will clear up on the face before the feet), recent symptoms will improve as older ones recur, and a long-term problem will improve (for example, asthma) as more superficial ones recur or are provoked (for example, eczema). There have been reports of some homeopaths advising their patients against vaccination and offering untested alternatives: well-qualified and experienced homeopaths do not agree with such advice.

Finding a homeopath

Anyone can set himself or herself up as a homeopath. But, while most homeopaths in the UK are not medically trained, the majority have had extensive training. To find a properly qualified lay homeopath, contact the Society of Homeopaths*: their 1,500 or so members undergo a three-year, full- or part-time training, have to follow strict codes and ethics, and are fully insured. RSHom after the name indicates that the practitioner is registered with the Society of Homeopaths, and FSHom that he or she is a Fellow of the Society of Homeopaths.

Homeopathy is also unique in complementary medicine in having a Faculty of Homeopathy* established by an Act of Parliament to train and register healthcare practitioners in homeopathy. The Faculty of Homeopathy promotes the academic and scientific development of homeopathy and regulates the education, training and practice of homeopathy by doctors, veterinary surgeons, podiatrists, dentists, nurses, midwives, pharmacists and other statutorily registered healthcare professionals. It now has over 1,300 members worldwide. There are about 1,000 doctors in the UK who practise homeopathy, usually alongside conventional medicine, of whom about 500 are registered with the Faculty. Around 230 of these doctors have completed basic training in a limited number of remedies for certain conditions and have the qualification FHom, while around 240 have a more in-depth training and the qualification MFHom.

Homeopathic remedies are also now widely available in pharmacies and health food shops to purchase for self-treatment. While convenient, there is a drawback with these off-the-shelf remedies – they are not specifically tailored to the individual and picking a remedy can be a bit hit-and-miss.

Hypnotherapy

Hypnotherapy is one of a wide range of techniques that come under the title of 'mind-body' medicine, a healing philosophy that recognises the profound link between the mind and body. In hypnotherapy, the therapist induces a hypnotic state, during which a person remains conscious but accepts suggestions more readily than usual, and acts on them more powerfully. Hypnotic practices can be traced back at least to the time of the ancient Egyptians, but Franz Anton Mesmer, a physician from Vienna, is generally regarded as being the founder of hypnotherapy as we know it today. He is reported to have successfully treated large numbers of people in the late eighteenth century by inducing deep trances. James Braid, a Scottish, Manchester-based surgeon, helped popularise hypnotism in the UK in the late nineteenth century and it was he who coined the term hypnotism (from the Greek word *hypnos*, meaning 'sleep'). However, it was not until the middle of the twentieth century that the conventional medical establishment began to accept that hypnotherapy could help in some situations.

How does hypnotherapy work?

Nobody is really sure how hypnotherapy works but one theory is that the left, analytical, side of the brain switches off during a hypnotic state, giving the right, creative, side a free rein. There is also much debate as to whether the hypnotic state is simply a state of deep relaxation or whether it represents an altered state of consciousness. Neither is it fully scientifically understood how hypnotic suggestions can enable people to deliberately control involuntary biological processes such as heart rate and skin temperature.

The aim of hypnotherapy is to enable a person to gain self-control over behaviour, emotions or biological processes. To achieve this, the hypnotherapist induces a hypnotic state in the patient. This state is said to be similar to being on 'automatic pilot'. It is not an end in itself but enables the person to accept and respond to suggestions from the therapist more readily. For example, in a treatment to stop smoking the hypnotherapist might suggest that you will no longer enjoy smoking or find it necessary. If you are in pain, the suggestion might be that the pain can be turned down like the volume of a radio. Once a person is hypnotised, he or she becomes absorbed in the message the hypnotherapist is giving but, most authorities agree, at all times, remains in control and cannot be made to do things he or she would not ordinarily agree to do. Some say that not everyone can enter a hypnotic state, but it is claimed that about 90 per cent of the population can be hypnotised to some degree and that 10 per cent can be taken into a hypnotic state so deep that they can tolerate minor operations without anaesthesia.

Who uses hypnotherapy?

Some people argue that hypnotherapy constitutes conventional medical treatment rather than complementary therapy. Others claim it is a form of psychotherapy; psychotherapists who use hypnotherapy are correctly described as hypno-psychotherapists, and deal with problems of mood, behaviour, thought or feeling. A medical doctor, unless also trained as a psychotherapist, helps with medical conditions. A number of doctors, dentists and clinical psychologists trained in hypnotherapy use hypnosis regularly and may offer it on the NHS. Hypnosis is also used in conjunction with cognitive behavioural therapy programmes in pain clinics or with occupational therapy in psychiatric units.

Hypnotherapy is most often used to treat pain, addictions, weight problems, phobias and fears, anxiety, depression, insomnia, medically unexplained symptoms (formerly known as psychosomatic conditions), asthma, eczema, allergies and irritable bowel syndrome.

Is it effective?

Hypnotherapy is supported by more scientific evidence than any other complementary therapy. Research into hypnosis can be divided into two types: basic research, which has focused on how hypnosis works; and clinical research, which has aimed at determining whether and for what hypnotherapy might be effective. A large number of clinical trials, and several systematic reviews, have been published, most of which appear to have originated in the USA and the UK. Some of the research has been of a high standard, but many trials have produced inconclusive results because they were too small, were not randomised or used inadequate control treatments.

A review of clinical trials of hypnotherapy for a wide range of problems found that there is reasonable evidence for its use for the treatment of asthma, skin conditions, irritable bowel syndrome, and to relieve nausea and vomiting during cancer treatment. In randomised controlled trials, hypnotherapy has been shown to improve relaxation in various medical conditions and prepare people for surgery, and to be helpful in controlling pain in children as well as adults. The results of a meta-analysis of 18 controlled trials suggest that hypnotherapy can enhance the effects of cognitive behavioural psychotherapy for a number of conditions, including anxiety, insomnia, pain and high blood pressure. Other studies suggest that hypnotherapy might help obese people to lose weight, help in the treatment of chronic fatigue syndrome and relieve headaches, improve conception in women with functional infertility and help bones to heal after a break. A systematic review has shown that it is no more effective than other interventions, or no treatment, for smoking cessation, although other research contradicts this finding.

A typical treatment

A hypnotherapist usually sees patients by themselves for between 30 and 90 minutes each session. In the initial session, you should be asked about your medical and family history and may be tested for hypnotic suggestibility. You may not necessarily be hypnotised in the first session. The therapist will then induce hypnosis using a variety of methods, which include speaking to you slowly and soothingly to help you relax, or asking you to look at lights or at a pencil held at the limits of your vision. The therapist will then probably ask you questions under hypnosis to find out the deeply rooted causes of your condition, and take you through procedures and suggestions to relieve it. You may be given direct hypnotic suggestion, for example, if you are scared of dental treatment you might be hypnotised during a dental procedure and given the suggestion that you are relaxed and calm. Most commonly, however, suggestions are made to a person in a hypnotic state that are aimed at altering behaviour or perception after the hypnosis has ended. For example, if you suffer from hay fever during the summer you might be told that you will no longer get symptoms when you come into contact with pollen. Your hypnotherapist might also help you to develop your ability to relax, to enable you to go into a deeply hypnotic state. You may also be taught techniques of self-hypnosis to manage your condition in your daily life. Some hypnotherapists carry out group hypnosis on ten or so patients at a time. This might be, for example, to teach self-hypnosis to a group of pregnant women to prepare them for labour. The average number of sessions needed to produce a result varies but is usually between six and 12, usually once a week. However, it is possible that just one may be enough. Each session may cost between £40 and £75 an hour.

How safe is it?

If a well-trained, experienced and regulated therapist carries it out, hypnotherapy should be safe. However, recovering repressed memories during hypnosis can be 'painful' and psychological problems may be exacerbated. There is some concern that hypnosis might trigger underlying psychosis, epileptic attacks or post-traumatic stress disorder. Although this has yet to be substantiated, caution needs to be exercised when using hypnosis in people with any of these conditions. There have been reports of false memories being introduced to people during hypnosis, which can lead to distress, cases of indecent assaults on people in a hypnotic state, and anecdotal reports of people not being returned fully to their pre-hypnotic state. However, no formal studies have been undertaken in an attempt to quantify these risks.

Finding a hypnotherapist

There are thousands of therapists practising hypnosis in the UK and anyone can set his or herself up as a hypnotherapist. Furthermore, there is no single regulating body, which can make it difficult to select an appropriate practitioner. Hypnotherapists with a conventional healthcare background, such as doctors, dentists, nurses and clinical psychologists, are regulated by their conventional professional regulatory bodies. However, there are several hundred hypnotherapists without such a background and they could be registered with one of several hypnotherapy registers. The training requirements, codes of conduct and disciplinary procedures of these different organisations vary widely. So, it is probably best to consult a clinically trained practitioner who only treats conditions within his or her own area of expertise. Hypnotherapy is not widely available on the NHS, but it might be possible to receive hypnotherapy on it through a conventionally trained healthcare professional who has also trained in hypnosis: for example, some dentists might offer it to people fearful of dental treatments or some pain clinics might offer it as a treatment for chronic pain.

Massage therapy

We all instinctively massage ourselves when we hurt something or have a pain, so massage has probably been around for as long as humans have. Paintings in Egyptian tombs show people being massaged, and ancient Chinese and Indian manuscripts refer to massage techniques to treat diseases. There are many different types of massage therapy. The most commonly used in the UK is classical (European or Swedish) massage, which first appeared in the late nineteenth century, when Per Henrik Ling, a Swedish gymnast, developed the principles of Swedish massage. The other main types of massage include Oriental massage such as marma (Indian), tuina (Chinese) and shiatsu (Japanese), and remedial and sports massage.

How does massage therapy work?

Massage therapy is the application of pressure to the soft tissues of the body – the skin, muscles, tendons and ligaments. Scientific trials investigating how massage might work have shown that it helps with relaxation generally, can increase your sense of well-being, helps muscles relax, increases blood flow locally and increases your pain threshold. The different types of massage utilise slightly different techniques: depending on the one used, a massage might relax, stimulate and/or strengthen the body.

Classical massage, developed by studying the anatomy of the body, comprises four main techniques. Effleurage, or stroking, is a smooth, gentle action where the hands glide rhythmically over the skin following the direction of the muscle fibres. It is used all over the body to relax tense muscles and improve circulation. Petrissage, or kneading of the skin and soft tissue by squeezing and releasing them, stretches and relaxes the muscles and is particularly used on fleshy areas. It helps to break up tension and scar tissue in the muscles. Frottage, or friction, involves applying deep pressure with the thumbs, knuckles or elbows to a specific spot to release tension in the muscles. Tapotement, percussion or chopping, with the sides of the hands, is used to stimulate the body and tone and strengthen the muscles.

Oriental types of massage tend to work on specific body points like acupuncture points and aim to move 'energy' in the body. **Shiatsu** is based on the same principles as Traditional Chinese Medicine and uses the same theories about Qi (known as Ki in Japanese) and meridians. The aims of shiatsu are to rebalance the recipient's 'energy' and treat conditions using pressure applied with the elbows, hands and fingers. This is believed to stimulate the body's own healing powers, get rid of toxins and promote general good health. Techniques used by a shiatsu practitioner may include gentle holding, pressing with the palms, thumbs, fingers, elbows, knees or feet on the meridians and, when appropriate, more dynamic rotations and stretches of the limbs and joints. Diagnosis in shiatsu is based on principles of oriental medicine as well as specific methods developed for shiatsu. **Tuina**, which is a traditional Chinese medical treatment, involves vigorous and deep techniques such as deep pressure on acupuncture points and kneading, squeezing and pushing to balance the flow of Qi in the meridians. Instead of using the flat of the hands, a tuina therapist pushes and twists into the flesh with the fingers, palms and knuckles – a vigorous but not uncomfortable procedure. Some people consider tuina a type of acupressure (see *Acupuncture*). **Marma** massage is a feature of Indian Ayurvedic medicine. Stimulating the marma points (similar to acupuncture points) is intended to encourage the flow of prana and bring about physical and mental well-being. Some massage therapists use aromatic oils during their treatments (see *Aromatherapy*).

Who uses massage therapy?

Today, massage is used for a wide range of reasons: for example, some people have it to help them wind down at the end of the working week, or to give their bodies a treat and lift; it is also increasingly used by various healthcare professionals. Physiotherapists practising within the NHS often use massage techniques and nine out of ten pain clinics in the UK have a massage practitioner. Many nurses are also now trained in massage and NHS-run hospitals, hospices, residential homes for older people, and units for those with learning disabilities or mental disorders also employ such nurses or massage therapists. It is less likely that you would be referred for massage therapy by your general practitioner, although some general practices do employ professional massage therapists. Many complementary therapists, such as acupuncturists, osteopaths and rolfers, also use massage techniques. Classical massage tends to be used predominantly in sports centres and health clubs; shiatsu and other Oriental-based massage therapies are used to treat a wide range of conditions from arthritis and migraines to digestive problems and asthma; remedial massage focuses on specific conditions such as minor soft-tissue injuries like muscle strains and joint sprains.

Is it effective?

In a survey published in *Which?* in December 2001, 71 per cent of respondents who had had massage therapy said they had been very satisfied, while 54 per cent said that it had greatly improved a specific health problem. There have been an increasing number of clinical trials in recent years looking at whether massage can result in clinical improvement in patients. Systematic reviews of such trials have found encouraging evidence that massage helps to relieve back pain, chronic constipation and pressure sores, but more studies are needed to confirm this. Several clinical trials have found that massage can help relieve anxiety and depression in people who are ill, such as young people with rheumatoid arthritis, children with cystic fibrosis, and patients being treated for cancer. They have also found that massage can reduce labour pain, help children with asthma breathe more easily, and help premature babies, heart and stroke patients, and people with AIDS, but more good-quality studies are needed. Although there is little scientific research to support the benefits of sports massage, a lot of anecdotal evidence suggests that it does improve recovery after hard exercise, help prevent injury and enhance performance. Little scientific research has been carried out on the Oriental-based massage therapies.

A typical treatment

It is important to make sure you pick the right kind of massage for you. To feel comfortable during your massage, avoid eating or drinking immediately before you have a massage, make sure you have emptied your bladder, and also tell your massage therapist if you feel cold or too warm during the treatment. As with most complementary therapies, a massage therapist will start off by asking you about your medical history, general state of health and perhaps your lifestyle. Oriental-based massage therapists may carry out a more detailed diagnosis, looking at your tongue, taking your pulses and palpating your muscles and abdomen, for any tender spots.

A classical massage can comprise a full body massage, with or without a facial massage, or just a neck and shoulder massage. For a full massage you will usually have to undress down to your underpants, although this is not compulsory. The therapist will then usually use towels to cover the parts of your body not being worked on. Classical massage therapists normally use an oil, or sometimes body lotion or talcum powder, to help their hands glide more easily over the skin. Shiatsu usually takes place on a padded mat or futon at floor level, although it is also possible to receive shiatsu sitting on a chair, if you are unable to lie down. For shiatsu, you can remain fully clothed but it is a good idea to wear loose, warm, comfortable clothing, preferably cotton, for example, a sweatshirt, tracksuit trousers and cotton socks. Shiatsu practitioners often teach their patients self-help exercises to maintain good health. Called 'do-in', these have elements of shiatsu and acupressure and comprise stretching exercises, tapping and pressure on acupressure points, breathing techniques and meditation. During a session of tuina, you also remain fully clothed and either sit on a chair or lie on a couch, depending on whether you are having your neck, arms, hands or back massaged. You will usually be given advice on diet and lifestyle. Oriental-based massage therapists may also encourage you to exercise regularly and make dietary changes.

How many massage sessions you need will depend on why you are having it. For help with a specific health or emotional problem, weekly sessions over a period of four to six weeks or longer may be needed; otherwise, one session a month is enough. The length of a classical massage session can vary, but a full-body massage usually takes about an hour, 1½ hours if the face is included. Other types of massage usually also take about an hour. A massage could cost anything from about £15 to £50, depending on the type, the length of the session and on where you are having it. The average cost of a massage is about £30.

How safe is it?

Massage is very safe when practised by a well-qualified therapist, but there are certain situations when it should not be used. You should not have a massage if you have a serious medical condition and should seek medical advice before having a massage if you have a blood clot (thrombosis), varicose veins or inflammation of the veins (phlebitis), a fever, acute arthritis, a severe back problem, an infective skin condition, cancer, HIV or AIDS, epilepsy or a serious psychiatric illness. Also, you should not be massaged on the abdomen, legs or feet during the first three months of pregnancy and it would be best to ask your doctor's advice about massage at other times during pregnancy. Shiatsu can be beneficial at any stage of pregnancy, provided that certain contra-indicated points – and the legs below the knee – are avoided. Massage should never be performed directly over bruises, or inflamed, infected or injured parts of the body. The pressure from some massage techniques can be temporarily uncomfortable. If any discomfort is unpleasant then ask the massage therapist to ease the pressure. You certainly should not feel persistent pain during a massage and, if you do, stop the treatment immediately. While you will usually experience a feeling of well-being, massage therapists claim that some people experience a 'healing' reaction after a massage, which could take the form of a headache or flu-like symptoms for 24 hours. You may also experience side-effects such as aches and pains for a day or two after a massage.

Finding a massage therapist

There are tens of thousands of massage therapists practising in the UK – anyone can set themselves up as a massage therapist without any training or regulation. Even if a therapist is trained, it can be difficult to know how good this training has been. Training can vary in length from a couple of weekends to a couple of years, and there are about 200 massage training schools and 60 massage qualifications. The danger is that some people who have only done a short course then set themselves up as being able to treat a wide range of heath problems, rather than simply using it to relax and soothe otherwise healthy people. If you have a serious condition, avoid having a massage that takes place in the 'health and beauty' context.

Also, be very wary of advertisements in newsagents and *Yellow Pages*: it takes little imagination to work out what is meant by 'executive massage' or 'exclusive services'.

The British Massage Therapy Council* can supply names of therapists who have done a basic minimum of 150 hours of tuition. The Massage Therapy Institute of Great Britain* holds the names of 600 practitioners. Some massage therapists may have qualifications from the International Therapy Examination Council (ITEC), which offers short basic courses in various therapies, including massage. Five hundred colleges now offer courses leading to ITEC qualifications. The Shiatsu Society* maintains a register of qualified practitioners, each of whom has been assessed for professionalism and clinical expertise by a panel of highly respected practitioners and teachers of shiatsu: members of the professional Register of the Shiatsu Society may use the initials MRSS. Continued use of the letters MRSS depends on maintaining current professional membership of the society, professional indemnity insurance, and a commitment to abide by the society's codes of ethics and conduct. The Shiatsu Society also maintains a list of graduates from its recognised schools who have not yet passed the MRSS assessment. Sports and remedial massage requires an understanding of the causes of injury, treatment, rehabilitation and training. Therapists with this level of training can be found through the Sports Massage Association*.

Naturopathy

Naturopathy is a complete approach to healthcare, which recognises that, given the right conditions, our bodies can cure themselves using innate vital forces. It developed out of the 'nature cures' that were used in Austrian and German health spas in the nineteenth century. Naturopaths believe that an unhealthy diet, the build-up of waste products in the body and a sedentary lifestyle are some of the main causes of illness. Naturopathic treatment aims to promote the body's ability to restore itself to good health and longevity. Naturopathy could be said to be more a way of life than a system of healthcare, and a great deal of emphasis is put on patient education and patient responsibility for staying healthy. Dietary measures are a central part of naturopathic treatment, as is hydrotherapy. However, naturopaths are often trained in other treatments as well, such as osteopathy or acupuncture.

How does naturopathy work?

An underlying principle of naturopathy is that our bodies are naturally self-regulating. This is known as the concept of homeostasis, which means that good health is the normal, harmonious state for human beings. Disease is generally thought to be due to a lack of harmony. For example, naturopaths believe that an unhealthy lifestyle and diet can overwhelm the body's natural self-regulating mechanisms and lead to illness. Naturopaths also believe that acute symptoms such as inflammation, fever or pain are signs that the body is working towards harmony again and that these symptoms should not be suppressed; for example, a high fever is thought to be produced in order to help our immunological defence mechanisms combat infection, so they would advise against using a drug to bring the temperature down. They also think that, during the process of recovery, the body might go through a healing crisis, during which symptoms get worse before getting better. Naturopathic treatments are directed at restoring the body to homeostasis by improving digestion and circulation, increasing the elimination of waste products and boosting the immune system.

Naturopaths believe that there are laws governing human function and our natural environment. The principle of vitalism states that every living thing has a vitality (life force), and that the existence of a healing power in nature (*vis medicatrix naturae*) means that our bodies can heal themselves because of their innate vitality. The triad of health recognises that there is a connection between the mind, body and spirit of all living beings, and that poor function in one part of the body inevitably leads to poor function elsewhere. The concept of individualism recognises that people are genetically, biochemically, structurally and emotionally different from one another. Naturopaths believe that we interact with our environment and that good health is a reflection of a harmonious interaction.

The defining elements of naturopathy are that it always: seeks to work with the body's own self-correcting mechanisms; attempts to address the mind, body and spirit; and regards health education as highly as treatment, so seeks to address lifestyle factors that are contributing to the problem and to re-educate the patient into a lifestyle more conducive to good health. The main principles of naturopathy are: first do no harm; prevention of a disease is better and easier than curing it; and it is important to treat the underlying causes of a patient's symptoms rather than the symptoms themselves.

Treatment can include advice about eating a wholefood diet rich in fresh fruit and vegetables (preferably organic), fasting, fresh air, vitamin and mineral supplements (see *Nutritional therapy*), herbal remedies, hydrotherapy, exercise and relaxation, as well as other complementary therapies. Hydrotherapy involves using both hot and cold water, steam and ice to prevent illness, boost vital energy, improve circulation and restore and cleanse the body. Baths, saunas, hot and cold compresses and wraps, whirlpools and water jets are all used. Seawater treatment (thalassotherapy) is also said to be healing.

Who uses naturopathy?

While naturopathic principles could be used to help with any health problem, they seem to be most suited to certain types of illness, including coughs and colds, sore throats and sinus problems, chronic conditions such as arthritis and asthma, skin problems, digestive disorders, general tiredness and chronic fatigue syndrome. The main uses of hydrotherapy are for arthritic problems, back pain, sports injuries, chest conditions, poor circulation, period problems, stress, headaches and chronic tiredness. In some states in the USA, naturopaths are licensed as GPs, and in Germany there are several thousand licensed naturopaths, or *Heilpraktikers*. In the UK, however, naturopathy is not widely available on the NHS, although elements are being increasingly integrated into the advice given by conventional healthcare professionals. As well as being widely used by naturopaths, hydrotherapy is an integral part of conventional medicine, where it is mainly used by physiotherapists.

Is it effective?

Conventional doctors now accept many of the beliefs of naturopathy and there is a wealth of evidence to support them; for instance, no one would question the benefits of the wholefood diet (rich in fibre and low in saturated animal fats) that it advocates, or that pesticides and chemical additives can be harmful to our health. Much of the naturopathic advice on vitamins and minerals has been backed up by scientific research too, although using mega-doses is still not supported by conventional medicine. As far as the non-dietary beliefs held by naturopaths are concerned, people all agree that lack of exercise and stress can lead to ill health. There have also been some individual clinical trials looking at the effects of fasting and hydrotherapy. Several studies have shown that controlled fasting can boost the immune system and general functioning of the body, while one trial found that taking a five-minute cold shower each morning for six months halved the number of colds participants suffered compared with those who took a warm shower. Evidence for other complementary therapies, such as acupuncture, herbal medicine, homeopathy, massage, osteopathy and relaxation, is relevant to naturopathy, as these are all therapies that a naturopath might use.

A typical treatment

Diagnosing what is wrong and why homeostasis has broken down is an important part of naturopathic treatment. So, on your first visit to a naturopath, which takes about an hour, you will be thoroughly questioned about your medical history, family history, symptoms, emotional well-being, lifestyle, diet, etc. Usually, you will have your blood, saliva and urine analysed to assess sugar, vitamin and mineral levels, and sometimes a sample of your hair will be sent away for analysis or you may be referred for X-rays. The naturopath will probably also look at your eyes (using iridology), skin, nails, mouth and tongue, listen to your heart and lungs with a stethoscope, take your blood pressure and feel your pulse. He or she may then carry out a physical examination of your joints and muscles to look for tenderness or joint stiffness. Naturopaths may also use diagnostic methods such as radionics/radiaethesia, applied kinesiology or Vega testing (see *Diagnostic alternatives*) to assess your vital energy. The naturopath will then use all the information gathered to assess how you are functioning overall and what your vital forces are like, as well as to diagnose what is wrong with you.

Essentially, the treatment you will be recommended will either be mainly anabolic (building up), if you are nutritionally deficient and have had your symptoms for some time, or catabolic (breaking down), if the problem seems to be due to a build-up of toxins. In either case, naturopathic treatment is as non-invasive as possible. Measures to build you up might include rest and relaxation, massage and gentle manipulation, a wholefood diet, and vitamin and mineral supplements. Measures to break down toxins might include elimination diets, fasting, hydrotherapy, colonic irrigation, and more vigorous exercise and manipulation. Dietary measures recommended by a naturopath might simply include increasing the amount of vitamin- and mineral-rich foods you eat, or might involve going on an elimination diet to try and identify foods that you are allergic to, or intolerant of, or might include detoxification through fasting. Given the right conditions, a fast is considered to be very beneficial and helps to restore good health. It is believed to give the body a rest and let it divert energy to the removal of toxins and to the restoring of harmony, rather than digesting and storing food. A fast can comprise eating only one food or one group of foods exclusively for a set amount of time: the most famous of this type of diet is the grape cure. It is inadvisable to fast without being supervised by a qualified practitioner. Naturopaths also recognise that poor body posture, misalignment of joints and muscle spasms can all affect health. Many are therefore trained in manipulative techniques such as osteopathy or chiropractic or they may recommend that you start practising the Alexander technique or yoga to realign your body. The role of emotions in ill health is considered very important by some naturopaths, who may spend some time counselling patients and some teach relaxation techniques, while others do not place much emphasis on the emotional status of the patient. Often, naturopathic treatment involves altering dietary and lifestyle habits over a long period of time, so it is only for the committed. After the initial consultation, you will probably need one or two follow-up appointments (lasting between 20 and 40 minutes) weekly for anything from a few weeks to several months, depending on how chronic or severe your condition is. However, the changes you make to your lifestyle and diet need to be lifelong to get the best benefits from them. The cost of a first naturopathy consultation can range from £35–£60 depending on your location, the follow-up sessions costing a little less. This does not include the cost of any herbal remedies or supplements that you are prescribed.

How safe is it?

The safety of naturopathy depends on the different therapies used (see relevant sections). Fasting can be dangerous in certain people, for example those with diabetes, and so it should be supervised. During a fast, the body releases toxins in the bloodstream and this can lead to people having headaches and feeling under the weather. Most naturopaths say this is a positive sign that the toxins are being eliminated and refer to it as a healing crisis.

Finding a naturopath

There are no laws regulating who can set him- or herself up as a naturopath. However, the General Council and Register of Naturopaths★ has a register of about 300 naturopaths practising in the UK. They have either taken a two-year part-time postgraduate course in naturopathy that is open to registered medical practitioners, osteopaths, chiropractors and medical herbalists and other practitioners trained in anatomy, physiology, pathology, diagnosis and clinical methods to primary healthcare levels, or will have completed the only four-year, full-time degree course in naturopathy that is available.

Nutritional therapy

Nutritional therapy, or nutritional medicine, is the use of diet and nutritional supplements as the main treatment for disease. Appreciation of the importance of what we eat and how it affects us probably dates back to ancient China, while Hippocrates recognised the importance of proper nutrition for good health and well-being. In recent years, nutritional therapy has grown in popularity as a specialisation of naturopathy. Nutrition is also part of conventional medicine, other complementary therapies include nutritional and dietary interventions, and Traditional Chinese Medicine and Ayurveda both have their own dietary theories.

How does nutritional therapy work?

Nutritional therapists believe that every illness involves an alteration in biochemistry, and that it is important to understand our biochemical make-up, how our nutritional status, diet and digestion can affect it, and what dietary and nutritional changes we can make to improve it. Interventions include nutritional supplements such as vitamins and minerals, food exclusion diets, and eating certain foods for medicinal purposes. Four main factors are considered by nutritional therapists to influence our nutritional status: the quality of the food we eat, the amount we eat, the efficiency of our digestive system, and each individual's biochemical make-up. Another aspect of nutritional therapy is food allergies and food intolerances, for which food-exclusion (elimination) diets are widely used. Finally, a more modern category of dietary supplements is probiotics: 'friendly' micro-organisms, such as lactobacillus, that are purported to maintain the health and balance of the gut flora. A popular theory in nutritional therapy is that a significant minority of us have a fungal infection (*Candida* or thrush) in our guts, which can result in symptoms such as bloating, diarrhoea, aching muscles and fatigue: proposed causes include antibiotics, oral contraceptives, steroid therapy, stress and chronic disease. Probiotics are given to help repopulate the gut with 'good' bacteria that we need to digest food properly. However, many conventional medical experts question the diagnosis of *Candida* in the gut as a common cause of symptoms.

Who uses nutritional therapy?

Nutritional therapists (see 'Finding a nutritional therapist' below for details) practise nutritional therapy. Practitioners of other forms of complementary medicine may also offer advice on diet.

Nutritional therapists commonly deal with a variety of different conditions, including asthma, sinusitis, skin conditions such as eczema, allergies, attention deficit hyperactivity disorder and sleep disturbances in children, migraine, headache, menstrual problems, cystitis, irritable bowel syndrome, obesity, fatigue, yeast (*Candida*) infections, auto-immune type conditions such as rheumatoid arthritis, and 'medically unexplained' symptoms. Nutritional therapists believe that a considerable proportion of 'healthy' people do not consume enough essential nutrients and that most of us would benefit from taking a general multivitamin and mineral supplement. Another aspect of nutritional therapy is the use of mega-doses of vitamins (see 'How safe is it?', below). This is called orthomolecular medicine.

In recent years, the value of nutritional advice has been increasingly recognised among conventional healthcare professionals as well. For example, doctors working in coronary care now recommend antioxidants such as vitamins A, C and E, while evening primrose oil containing gamma-linolenic acid is considered an effective conventional treatment for cyclical mastalgia (breast pain associated with the menstrual cycle).

Is it effective?

In April 2000 *Health Which?* published research it had carried out to look at the quality of advice given by nutritional therapists. It showed that there was a lack of consistency in performance, for example, inadequate history-taking, recommendations of inappropriate products, and a lack of advice to see a GP.

There is a wealth of scientific research to show that certain diets can increase our risk of developing heart disease, having a stroke or getting certain cancers. Numerous studies have been published about nutritional influences on health and illness, and there are some clinical trials supporting the use of nutritional supplements to improve health, prevent disease and treat specific diseases. And, of course, for many people one of the biggest benefits of a healthy diet is weight loss: after all, obesity is one of the biggest health problems in the industrialised world and increases your risk of getting heart disease, diabetes, certain cancers and arthritis.

Randomised controlled trials have shown that individual supplements may help: for example, zinc supplements may help to treat the common cold, glucosamine and chondroitin have been shown to help relieve the pain of arthritis, and calcium and vitamin D supplements can help to prevent osteoporosis. The benefits of a low-fat, high-fibre diet rich in fruit and vegetables are well known and this diet is widely advocated by healthcare professionals from all backgrounds. Trial results also suggest that antioxidants (for example, vitamins A, C and E) may protect against premature ageing, cancer and heart disease, and that they may also be beneficial in arthritis and asthma, although other research contradicts this. Free radicals work by finding and mopping up free radicals in the body – these are molecules that our bodies make as part of the defence against bacteria. Free radical levels can also be increased owing to cigarette smoke, chemicals and industrial pollution. Although free radicals only 'live' for a few seconds, they can damage DNA (genetic material) in cells and affect cholesterol so that it is more likely to stick to artery walls. These actions may make us more susceptible to cancer and to heart and circulatory disorders.

A typical session

At your first appointment with a nutritional therapist, which will last about an hour, you should be asked about your health and symptoms, your medical and family history, and your emotional state, diet and lifestyle. Many therapists use dietary questionnaires to find out if you have any nutritional deficiencies or food intolerances. Some nutritional therapists also assess your skin, eyes, tongue, nails and reflexes, and some may take a hair sample for mineral analysis, use iridology, Vega testing or applied kinesiology and possibly blood, sweat, stool and urine samples. The nutritional therapist will then give you a combination of vitamins, minerals and other supplements tailored specifically for you. Some nutritionists also use medicinal herbs. You may also be prescribed a specific diet, such as a vegetarian diet (no meat or fish), a raw food diet, a detoxification diet, the Hay or food-combining diet (eating protein and carbohydrates at different meals) or vegan diet (no meat, fish, eggs, dairy or honey). The cost of a first nutritional therapy session is abut £25–£85, depending on your location. Follow-up sessions take about 15–20 minutes and cost between £15 and £50. You will probably need several sessions, depending on your condition and how long you have had it. Supplements and other products can also increase the costs.

How safe is it?

High doses of vitamins can cause side-effects: for example, high doses of vitamin C can cause diarrhoea, while high doses of vitamin B6 can cause peripheral neuropathy, and the oil-soluble vitamins A and D can result in serious side-effects if they are taken in high doses as they accumulate in the body. With minerals, high doses of magnesium can cause low blood pressure and flushing, and high doses of potassium and selenium are toxic. The Expert Group on Vitamins and Minerals (EGVM), which was set up by the government, is systematically reviewing what are 'safe' levels of vitamin and mineral supplements. Also, European Union legislation to limit the levels of vitamins and minerals that can be added to supplements, based on the establishment of safe upper limits by the EU's Scientific Committee for Food, was imminent as this book went to press.

Children, pregnant and lactating women, and patients with chronic illness should only make major dietary changes under professional supervision. Also, always check with your doctor before you start taking nutritional supplements if you are taking any medication (conventional or otherwise), as they may interact.

Finding a nutritional therapist

In the UK anyone can call him- or herself a nutritional therapist, even if he or she has had only minimal training; training for nutritional therapy can vary from short correspondence courses leading to a certificate in basic nutrition to full-time university BSc degree courses leading to a qualification as a nutritional therapist. However, the British Association of Nutritional Therapists★ (BANT), a voluntary professional body which holds a register of about 200 nutritional therapists, has set interim standards for its members until new national standards are set for all therapists. BANT says that unless a nutritional therapist has medical training he or she should not diagnose a medical condition. BANT registers practitioners who have completed one of its approved courses at selected training colleges. The British Society for Allergy and Environmental Medicine and Nutritional Medicine★ is an association of British doctors who are interested in the use of nutrition in clinical medicine. Education in nutrition is also increasingly being taught as part of the undergraduate medical curriculum. You can also get dietary advice on the NHS from state-registered dieticians (SRD), who are listed by the British Dietetic Association★. SRDs have degrees in nutritional science and are registered by law. They also practise outside the NHS. Registered nutritionists (RN) also have degrees, but do not generally provide therapeutic advice direct to members of the public.

Osteopathy

Osteopathy is a manipulation-based therapy that comprises a recognised system of diagnosis and treatment. It has its roots as far back as Hippocrates in 400BC, but the US doctor Andrew Taylor Still, who formalised osteopathic treatment in the late nineteenth century, is considered to be the founder of osteopathy. He believed that many health problems can be traced to disorders of the muscles and joints, particularly the spine, and that if the structure of the body is improved its function improves too. The first school of osteopathy in the UK was in London in 1917. Today, in the UK, there are around 3,000 osteopaths, who perform over six million patient consultations a year. Osteopathy has much in common with chiropractic, but there are also differences between the two. While chiropractors lay more emphasis on the joints of the spine, osteopaths lay equal emphasis on the joints and surrounding soft tissue (ligaments and muscles). The word osteopathy derives from the Greek words *osteon*, meaning 'bone', and *pathos*, meaning 'disease'.

How does osteopathy work?

The way osteopathy works is not fully understood scientifically. Osteopaths believe that the body is self-healing, and when the musculoskeletal system is out of balance, this can affect the organs which are supported and protected by it. The musculoskeletal system is the largest system of the body and an imbalance in it is thought to cause much of the pain and ill health we suffer. Imbalance is said to arise because of physical or emotional stress, injury or poor posture, which can be sport-, leisure-, or work-related. Another important factor can be problems arising during development. For example, if one leg is shorter than the other, this can lead to curvatures of the spine, which can subsequently affect the efficiency of the respiratory and cardiovascular systems.

An osteopath uses a wide range of techniques to ensure perfect alignment in the body, including: high-velocity, low-amplitude thrusts (short, rapid, forceful movements to spinal joints to extend them slightly); muscle energy techniques (when muscle tension is released by working against resistance provided by the osteopath); gentle massage; rhythmic joint movements; and lymphatic pump techniques (designed to improve lymphatic drainage). When a high velocity thrust is performed, you may hear a loud and rather unnerving click. This is said to be caused by gas bubbles in the synovial fluid. A bubble forms within the joint and then disperses in a fraction of a second when the high-velocity thrust is applied.

Who uses osteopathy?

The main aim of osteopathy is to reduce pain, inflammation and immobility by restoring optimum function of the musculoskeletal system. The most common problems treated by osteopaths are neck and back pain, as well as pain in other parts of the body that are due to problems in the spine, such as migraine or facial pain. Osteopathy is also used to treat other structurally related problems, such as changes to posture in pregnancy, repetitive strain injury, the pain of arthritis and sports injuries. Many osteopaths see their role as wider than treating just the immediate problem, and will treat other conditions that do not seem obviously related to problems with the structure of the body, such as breathing problems and menstrual disorders. Cranial osteopathy and craniosacral therapy are used widely for treating babies with colic, sleeplessness and feeding problems, or when they have had a difficult birth (for example, a Caesarean birth or when interventions such as forceps or suction have been used).

Most people consult an osteopath privately, but an increasing number of osteopaths also work with GP practices. It is also possible for your doctor to refer you to an osteopath on the NHS: about a third of GPs in the UK refer patients for osteopathy. The current guidelines from the Royal College of General Practitioners recommend that manipulative treatment to improve movement in someone with low back pain should be considered, if the person still has pain or if they have not returned to ordinary activity or work within six weeks of the symptoms starting. Many private health insurance schemes provide benefit for osteopathic treatment, either reimbursing the total fee or paying a percentage of the costs. Contact the helpline of your insurance company to find out the actual benefits and methods of claim for your individual policy.

Is it effective?

In a survey published in *Which?* in December 2001, 69 per cent of respondents who had had osteopathy said they had been very satisfied, while 66 per cent said that it had greatly improved a specific health problem. There are very few clinical trials that expressly look at osteopathy, but there is some evidence to suggest that osteopathy is helpful for low back pain, particularly in the acute and sub-acute stages. Little has been done to compare osteopathy with other manipulative treatments such as chiropractic. There have been several systematic reviews of clinical trials investigating spinal manipulation and mobilisation for low back pain; however, many of the trials included in these reviews are of questionable quality and the research does not show how many treatments are needed to achieve maximum benefit. A recent review, which analysed the best evidence available, suggested that spinal manipulation (whether done by an osteopath, chiropractor, physiotherapist or doctor) is effective in the short term for acute low back pain. It also found it to be effective for chronic low back pain when compared with placebo and commonly used treatments such as those used by GPs, but found that the evidence was inconclusive for mixed acute and chronic low back pain and for sciatica. There are fewer trials of manipulation and mobilisation techniques for neck pain and the results of these trials vary. A recent systematic review of osteopathy in other conditions found no compelling evidence that it was effective. There has been very little clinical research on cranial osteopathy (see below).

A typical treatment

An osteopath will usually see patients for about 60 minutes at the first session and about 20–30 minutes at subsequent sessions. At the first session you will be asked your medical history and the osteopath will also carry out a careful physical examination, and observe you standing, walking and sitting. You will normally be asked to remove some of your clothing and to perform a simple series of movements. The osteopath will then use a highly developed sense of touch, called palpation, to identify any points of weakness or excessive strain in your body. Sometimes an osteopath may take your blood pressure, test your reflexes or arrange for you to have an X-ray or blood tests. Your treatment will then be tailored to your individual needs. You will usually be treated lying down, although some manipulation may be carried out while you are sitting or standing. Osteopaths usually start any treatment by releasing and relaxing muscles and stretching stiff joints and, while they do carry out spinal manipulations, they form a much smaller part of treatment than in chiropractic. For children and older people, in particular, they may use only gentle 'release techniques' rather than manipulations. Osteopaths may also carry out cranial manipulation (cranial osteopathy, and the related craniosacral therapy), which involves gentle palpation of the bones of the skull and back. This is aimed at correcting disturbances in the flow of cerebrospinal fluid, which are said to reflect injuries or tension in the body. Your osteopath may show you exercises to do at home and suggest ways you can improve your posture. Some osteopaths also give nutritional advice. The number of treatments needed depends on your condition. If you have low back pain, for example, you might need around six weekly treatments. For some acute pain, one or two treatments may be all that is necessary. The cost of a first session ranges from £30–£70 and for subsequent sessions from £20–£50.

How safe is it?

After an osteopathic treatment, you may feel stiff or sore for a few hours, which can be helped by mild painkillers. The pain usually subsides within 24 hours of the treatment. You might also experience a slight headache or tiredness. The most serious potential adverse effects with osteopathy are stroke and spinal cord injury after manipulation. However, while the risk of such events has not been quantified, it is believed to be extremely rare. Osteopaths normally use less forceful techniques than chiropractors (such as spinal mobilisation rather than manipulation), so it seems likely that osteopathy is less risky in terms of spinal trauma, although no data are available to verify this. People who have certain conditions –

such as osteoporosis, rheumatoid arthritis, recent fractures and whiplash injuries – should not be subject to forceful manipulation. Osteopaths are highly trained to screen patients for these and other risk factors. However, even with careful screening there is always the possibility of a person having an undetectable underlying condition. If you do have one of these conditions, other more gentle manipulative treatments, such as cranial osteopathy, may be safer.

Finding an osteopath

In the UK, osteopaths are regulated by legal statute and it is illegal for people to call themselves an osteopath unless they are on the Statutory Register of the General Osteopathic Council (GOsC)★. The GOsC was established after the Osteopaths Act was passed by Parliament in 1993, and has similar powers to the General Medical Council (GMC)★ in that it can remove practitioners from its register after a disciplinary hearing. There are now over 3,000 osteopaths registered in the UK, all of whom have undergone at least four years of full-time (or six years of part-time) training at a recognised college; are covered by professional indemnity insurance; are bound by a strict and enforceable code of practice; and have to take part in postgraduate training. It is also possible for doctors to complete fast-track training in osteopathy on a 12–18-month course. Those practitioners registered after 1993 have shown that they are safe and competent practitioners through a revalidation process.

Reflexology

Reflexology, sometimes called reflex zone therapy or zone therapy, involves applying pressure to certain areas on the feet and, less often, the hands. The aim with reflexology is to treat the whole person and help the body heal itself by restoring and maintaining balance in the body. Some reflexologists also believe that reflexology can be used diagnostically (see page 181). The oldest reference to reflexology comes from pictures in the tomb of an ancient Egyptian physician dating from about 2400BC. There is also evidence that foot massage and reflexology in some form or other was used by early African tribes, native Americans and in ancient China and India. However, reflexology as we know it today owes its revival to an ear, nose and throat surgeon, Dr William Fitzgerald, in the early twentieth century. He discovered that he could anaesthetise one part of the body by applying pressure to a certain part of the foot, and developed the theory that the body is divided into ten vertical zones running from the feet to the head and out to the hands and vice versa. He claimed that 'energy' flows through these zones and that, when there is an imbalance in the energy somewhere in the body, there is a change of texture (a crystalline deposit forms at the relevant reflex point on the foot or hand), causing a blockage in the energy flow. Applying pressure on these areas allows the energy to flow freely again and so promotes good health and well-being. A few years later, a massage therapist, Eunice Ingham, created the foot reflexology maps as we know them today (see pages 152 and 153). Reflexology was introduced to the UK in 1968 by a student of Ingham's, Doreen Bayley, who set up the first UK school of reflexology (the Bayley School).

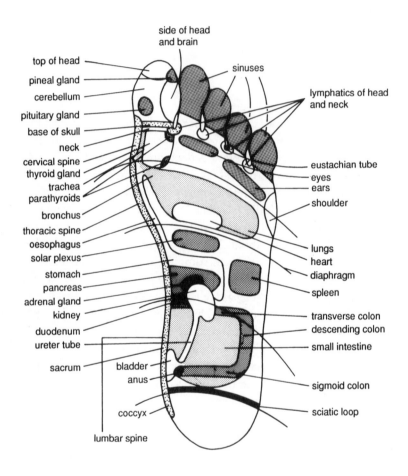

top of head
pineal gland
cerebellum
pituitary gland
base of skull
neck
cervical spine
thyroid gland
trachea
parathyroids
bronchus
thoracic spine
oesophagus
solar plexus
stomach
pancreas
adrenal gland
kidney
duodenum
ureter tube
sacrum
bladder
anus
coccyx
lumbar spine

side of head
and brain
sinuses

lymphatics of head
and neck

eustachian tube
eyes
ears
shoulder

lungs
heart
diaphragm
spleen

transverse colon
descending colon
small intestine

sigmoid colon

sciatic loop

The reflexes on the left foot as seen from underneath

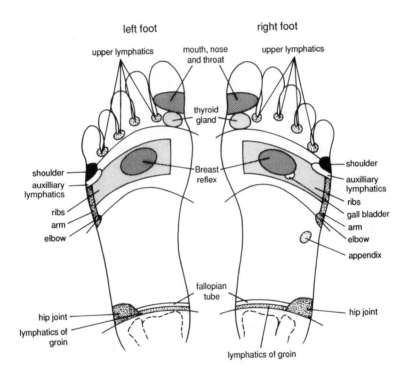

The reflexes on top of the feet

How does reflexology work?

Reflexologists believe that the reflex zones on the feet and hands correspond to zones in the body. The zones on the right foot correspond to the right side of the body and those on the left foot to the left side, and an imaginary line drawn halfway down across the foot corresponds to the waistline, with the big toes representing the head and brain, the sole as the abdominal area and the heels as the pelvic region. Because all parts of the body are represented on the feet (and hands), the whole body can be treated in a session. Alternatively, just the affected part of the body can be treated by focusing on the zones for that area. Applying pressure to the points is said to free up any energy blockages in the zones of the body, and so help to relieve stress, and to prevent or treat ill health. Some people believe that reflexology is related to acupuncture: this might be the case, but there is currently no scientific evidence linking them. However, auricular (ear) acupuncture and Korean hand acupuncture are based on similar concepts to reflexology. It is now quite common for complementary therapists who practise massage, aromatherapy and other body therapies to also offer reflexology.

Who uses reflexology?

Reflexology is used to relieve stress, improve circulation, prevent ill health by eliminating toxins, treat a range of physical disorders and sometimes to diagnose disease (see page 181). The conditions it might be used for include anxiety and insomnia, back and neck pain, period problems, menopausal symptoms, skin conditions, asthma, sinus problems, high blood pressure, digestive problems, migraine and headaches. Although reflexology is not widely available on the NHS, many nurses, midwives and physiotherapists have trained in reflexology, and an increasing number of reflexologists are being employed in NHS hospitals.

Is it effective?

In a survey published in *Which?* in December 2001, 73 per cent of respondents who had had reflexology said they had been very satisfied, while 42 per cent said that it had greatly improved a specific health problem. There is no scientific evidence to confirm the existence of the reflex zones, energy lines or crystalline deposits (for example, there are no known connections, such as via nerves, between the reflex zones on the feet and the organs or glands in the body). However, there are some 7,000 nerve endings in each foot, so it is possible that pressing on these could induce feelings of deep relaxation. The quality of scientific studies testing the effectiveness of reflexology has generally been poor, but this does not mean that reflexology has no health benefits. Indeed, there is some evidence from randomised placebo-controlled trials that it: may help with pre-menstrual symptoms; can reduce anxiety; may help relieve symptoms of multiple sclerosis; and may benefit people with diabetes. However, a review of the results of several scientific studies evaluating reflexology concluded that, overall, it has not been shown to be any more effective than placebo treatment. Regardless of the scientific evidence, or lack of it, for a benefit with reflexology, anecdotally people report feeling very relaxed after a reflexology treatment.

A typical treatment

At your first appointment with a reflexologist, you will usually be asked about your medical history and lifestyle, whether you are taking any medication and whether you have come to be treated for a specific condition. During the treatment, you will be asked either to lie down or sit on a reclining chair with your feet raised. Do not worry if your feet are hot and sweaty, as the practitioner will wipe them before starting. The therapist will work on your feet, or some-times your hands if necessary, for example, if you have a health problem (for example, gout, ulceration) that that affects your feet. A treatment lasts between 30 minutes and one hour. Reflexologists use their hands, and particularly their thumbs, first to examine your feet and then to give the treatment. Gentle massage is used to start with, followed by deep pressure. The therapist may use talcum powder or oil to lubricate your feet and some add specific essential oils (as used in aromatherapy) to the base oil. You may feel some discomfort or tenderness during the treatment, but this should be brief. On the whole, the feelings you experience during a reflexology session should be relaxing and pleasant. The number of treatments someone needs varies depending on the individual and his or her situation, but the average length of a course is 6–8 treatments. The cost of treatment can range from £25–£40, depending on your location.

How safe is it?

In the hands of a well-trained and responsible therapist, reflexology seems to be safe, although its safety has not been evaluated in rigorous scientific studies. The side-effects of reflexology seem to be mild and short-lasting, such as slight pain and tenderness on the feet during the treatment itself, and brief changes in bowel or bladder function, such as wanting to go to the lavatory more often than usual. People have also reported feeling sick, 'fluey', sleepy or weepy after a session. These are described as healing reactions when toxins are being released and eliminated from the body. If you are pregnant, or have a heart or circulatory problem, thrombosis (blood clot), a thyroid disorder, epilepsy, depression or diabetes, you should consult with your doctor first to see whether reflexology is appropriate for you. If you are on any medication, conventional or otherwise, it is important to tell your reflexologist, as reflexology can increase your body's elimination processes, which could reduce the effectiveness of any medication you are taking. Also, essential oils, if used, can themselves cause side-effects (see page 84).

One of the most worrying risks with reflexology is its use as a diagnostic tool (see page 181), as this could lead to unnecessary medical treatment or, worse, no treatment when it is vital. All professional reflexology associations insist that their members do not claim to be able to diagnose disease and, if a reflexologist suspects from an assessment of your feet that there may be a serious underlying condition, he or she should advise you to go to your GP. However, there have been a few reports of reflexologists making false positive or negative diagnoses. The Reflexology Forum (see below) states that it is against the codes of practice and ethics of all its member organisations to make any medical diagnoses.

Finding a reflexologist

There are no legal requirements for the practice of reflexology and anyone can set himself or herself up as a reflexologist, without any training at all. However, there are at least ten reflexology organisations in the UK that require their members, to a greater or lesser degree, to be trained: around 13,000 reflexologists now belong to one or other of these organisations. The Reflexology Forum★, representing all the major UK organisations, has recently been set up with the aim of achieving high standards of training and practice and also self-regulation. The Association of Reflexologists★ has accredited nearly 80 courses in the UK which meet its standards. The British Reflexology Association★ is the professional organisation associated with the Bayley School. Both organisations have codes of practice and ethics, and therapists must have insurance. The International Federation of Reflexologists★ is the largest reflexology membership body, with some 8,500 names on its register.

Relaxation and meditation

True relaxation occurs when the mind is still, the muscles deeply relaxed and the breathing regular and slow. There are several techniques that can help you relax in this way, such as meditation, deep breathing and muscle relaxation, and all of them can be mastered quite easily with a little practice. Meditation has been part of most spiritual practices from Buddhism and Hinduism to Christianity and Judaism for centuries, while yoga uses breathing to bring about inner peace. It is, however, only relatively recently that researchers have discovered the therapeutic benefits of relaxation and meditation.

Other complementary therapies, such as autogenic therapy, biofeedback, hypnotherapy, visualisation and yoga also induce deep relaxation, and together these therapies come under the umbrella of mind-body medicine.

How do relaxation and meditation work?

Stress triggers the body's 'fight or flight' response, an instinctive reaction to acute stress, such as a life-threatening event, and is a throwback to our primitive roots to get our bodies ready to fight or run away from a predator or enemy. Several hormones are released into the bloodstream in response to acute stress, such as adrenaline and noradrenaline. These make the heart beat stronger and faster, and our breathing become rapid and shallow, so that more oxygen flows to the brain to increase alertness and to the muscles, so that they contract in readiness for action. At the same time, blood flow is reduced to other parts of the body that are not involved in the need to survive the emergency, such as the digestive tract and skin. It is as if the body is on red alert, and so when we are under chronic stress, our bodies are on constant red alert, which can lead to physical and emotional symptoms. Calming the mind and relaxing the body using relaxation techniques or meditation can break this constant 'fight or flight' response.

Breathing is automatic and we do not usually exert any control over it. However, we can consciously control our breathing and this can form a useful bridge between our bodies and our minds. Deep abdominal breathing means exactly what it sounds like, breathing deeply into the abdomen. Many of us are what is known as chest breathers, that is, we only breathe into our upper chest and lungs as if we are under acute stress. This may lead to 'overbreathing' and so to an imbalance of oxygen and carbon dioxide in the blood, which can result in many of the symptoms characteristic of stress, such as headache, insomnia, panic attacks and palpitations. It is considered to be more healthy to breathe into your abdomen and consciously doing deep abdominal breathing, sometimes called diaphragmatic breathing, can help you to relax, as well as train you to breathe into your abdomen all the time.

When we are under stress, the muscles become tense, which can result in pain and fatigue. Consciously trying to relax your muscles is an effective way of relaxing the body and will also calm the mind. Deep muscle relaxation involves tensing all the muscles in your body at the same time and then letting them go. Progressive muscle relaxation is similar to deep muscle relaxation but involves tensing and relaxing one muscle group at a time.

Meditation can be broadly defined as any activity that keeps the mind calm, clear of all thoughts and focused on the present. While it is practised as a way of reaching spiritual enlightenment in Eastern societies, it can be practised outside of a religious or philosophical context as a useful self-help technique. It essentially involves either focusing on something such as your breath, a mantra (for example, Om) or an object (for example, a candle flame), or being aware of your thoughts but not engaging in them.

Who uses relaxation and meditation?

Relaxation techniques and meditation are used by a wide range of people, for many different reasons. Some people meditate for spiritual reasons, others to relieve stress and improve well-being. Relaxation techniques and meditation are also used to treat specific conditions, particularly those that are triggered or made worse by stress, such as high blood pressure, anxiety, insomnia, phobias, asthma, eczema, pain, menstrual and menopausal problems, and irritable bowel syndrome. Healthcare professionals are increasingly recognising the value of relaxation techniques and meditation and they are often taught in NHS hospitals, for example, on coronary care units or in psychiatric units, and in health centres. Many complementary practitioners also use relaxation methods and meditation with their patients, as do psychotherapists and clinical psychologists.

In the UK, three types of meditation are widely practised. **Transcendental meditation (TM)★**, which is practised by around 200,000 people in the UK, is used predominantly to alleviate stress and is gaining acceptance in medical circles. It involves spending 20 minutes twice a day sitting comfortably with your eyes closed and silently repeating a special word or mantra. The British Association for the Medical Application of Transcendental Meditation has a membership of 700 GPs and hospital doctors, who are campaigning for TM on the NHS. **Buddhist meditation** practices involve developing awareness of breathing and of positive feelings for all living beings, in an attempt to achieve inner peace and calm. **Vedic mantra meditation** as taught by the School of Meditation★ in London is a technique that allows the attention to rest on a simple sound to which you attach no attitude or emotions. This gives access to the deeper, still part of the mind.

Are they effective?

Muscle relaxation has been shown scientifically to normalise blood supply to the muscles, reduce oxygen use, slow the heartbeat and breathing and reduce muscle activity. It also increases alpha brainwaves and skin resistance, which are a sign of relaxation. Other relaxation techniques have been shown to be effective in reducing muscle tension. Meditation also leads to the production of alpha brainwaves and changes in muscle tone and skin resistance. There is some evidence that it may boost the neurotransmitter serotonin, in the same way as an antidepressant drug but without the side-effects.

There is much good scientific evidence to show that relaxation therapies can help reduce anxiety. Randomised controlled trials have shown that relaxation can also help with agoraphobia, panic disorder and anxiety associated with serious medical conditions such as cancer. The evidence for a beneficial effect on acute or chronic pain is less clear; the trials have often been of poor quality and the results have been contradictory. There is, however, promising evidence from randomised controlled trials looking at relaxation for depression, insomnia, migraine, high blood pressure, asthma and menopausal symptoms.

Most of the studies attesting to the benefits of meditation relate to TM. Some 500 scientific studies on TM have been published since the mid-1970s, all testifying to the effectiveness of this form of meditation in the treatment of anxiety, mild depression, insomnia, tension headaches, migraine, high blood pressure, irritable bowel syndrome, post-natal depression and a number of stress-related conditions. Some of this research has been published in journals that do not require a rigorous peer review or has been reviewed by other people in the TM organisation, so it may lack objectivity. However, clinically based trials in peer-reviewed journals have shown TM to lower blood pressure in people with hypertension, reduce artherosclerosis in the heart's blood vessels, and decrease anxiety. The few studies comparing TM with other forms of meditation have conflicting results.

A typical session

It can be difficult for a beginner to learn how to relax or to still the mind with meditation, so a teacher and the discipline of being in a group can be invaluable. Typically, a relaxation technique or meditation may be learnt over a course of 5–10 sessions and you will also be encouraged to practise what you have learnt daily at home. Practitioners of relaxation techniques or meditation do not make a diagnosis, but may ask you about your health problems, so as to be able to tailor a relaxation programme for you.

Some types of relaxation or meditation can be practised almost anywhere. However, complete relaxation is more likely to be achieved in calm surroundings, with low lighting and a minimum of noise (except perhaps some gentle music or a guided-relaxation tape) and activity. You can relax or meditate lying down, sitting or standing up. For relaxation, it is probably best to lie down, while sitting is probably best for meditation, either on an upright chair or on a cushion on the floor with your back against the wall, because standing is tiring, and it is easy to fall asleep when lying down.

Whatever position you choose, it is important to find a position that you will be comfortable in for about 15–20 minutes, the length of time you will be advised to practise on a daily basis. Meditation is more effective, the stiller you stay.

Training in relaxation is usually free on the NHS; privately, it varies in cost depending on your location and whether you are learning it as part of a group or individually. Some fundholding GPs prescribe TM under the NHS, but this is rare. A course of TM normally costs around £500 (£400 for students). A six-week course in Buddhist meditation, consisting of 2½ hours of tuition a week, costs around £60 (£40 for unwaged people), while for a week's meditation retreat you might pay £350 (£250 if unwaged). The School of Meditation requests a one-off donation of one week's income for the teaching of the technique and all subsequent guidance. Students, the unwaged and the over-60s are asked to give £100.

How safe are they?

Both relaxation techniques and meditation are probably best avoided by people with schizophrenia or psychosis, at least without medical supervision. Although effective meditation brings about mental and emotional calm, if you meditate without the support of a trained and experienced teacher, worries and fears may surface that can provoke more stress and may even do harm. Those who are most vulnerable are people who do not face up to what is happening in their lives. People who meditate regularly, and with support, admit that although painful memories may surface, meditation itself equips one with enough emotional and mental strength to deal with them.

Finding a teacher

There is a complete lack of regulation in this field but, given the relative safety of relaxation techniques and meditation, this is unlikely to be harmful. Rather, it presents more of a problem of making sure that you receive effective tuition for a reasonable price. Training in how to teach relaxation techniques or meditation varies enormously from weekend courses to apprenticeships that can last for several years (for example, Buddhist monks). TM is taught in 50 centres across the UK. It is advisable to go to an introductory lecture before deciding to enrol in the training, which is expensive. If you decide that TM is for you, you will probably attend four sessions on consecutive days and a further session three months later. Buddhist meditation is taught by teachers in Buddhist centres across the UK. The Friends of the Western Buddhist Order (FWBO)* runs meditation classes in more than 20 permanent centres and short retreats in rural centres in the UK. Other Buddhist organisations run centres too. The School of Meditation* in London holds introductory meetings or private interviews. Instruction in mantra meditation is given at a later date, on an individual basis, in a session lasting 90 minutes. Individual guidance is available after the initial instruction for as long as a member needs it. Group studies of the tradition (Vedic) from which this meditation technique comes are run throughout the year.

Yoga

Classical yoga is a complete system, or way of life. The word 'yoga' means union, and comes from the Sanskrit word *yuj*, which translates as 'to yoke' or 'to balance'. In the East, yoga is a way of working towards self-awareness, personal development and spiritual enlightenment, but it does not need to be an all-consuming spiritual practice. In fact, in the West, yoga is often valued more for its physical benefits than its spiritual ones and is usually taken to mean the practice of yoga postures, yoga breathing and meditation as a way of improving physical and mental well-being. Yoga originated in India several thousand years ago, and the philosophy of yoga was first ordered and written down at least 2,000 years ago by a sage called Patanjali. His work is known as the *Yoga Sutra* and is still considered among the most authoritative writing on yoga. Yoga first reached the West in the 1890s but really took off in the 1950s, when Swami Sivananda, one of the great Indian yoga practitioners of the time, sent his disciple Swami Vishnudevananda to the West to spread the knowledge and practice of yoga.

How does yoga work?

Yoga is a philosophy, a science and an art, as well as a therapy. Classical yoga, as practised in the East, is organised into eight limbs, or parts, which together affect every aspect of life: Yama, or universal ethics for right living; Niyama, or personal discipline; Asanas, or the yoga postures; Pranayama, or yoga breathing; Pratyahara, or withdrawing the senses from the external world; Dharana, or the concentration of the mind; Dhyana, or meditation; Samadhi, or enlightenment or the state of bliss and 'truth'. These eight limbs are a progressive series of steps said to purify mind and body, each of the limbs growing simultaneously to achieve this. However, even practising only certain of the limbs of yoga, such as the postures (asanas) or the breathing (pranayama), is considered more beneficial than simply exercising, as it involves the mind as well as the body. It is like a moving meditation because, as your mind concentrates on what your body is doing, it becomes focused and calm. Yoga is also said to improve the flow of prana (the life force, which is the equivalent of Qi in the Chinese tradition). The chakras are a series of seven prana centres that lie along the midline of the body. They include the crown chakra at the top of the head, the brow chakra between the eyebrows, the throat chakra just in front of the voice box, the heart chakra halfway along the sternum, the solar plexus chakra midway between the bottom of the sternum and the belly button, the sacral chakra just below the belly button, and the base chakra at the centre of the perineum. Each chakra is said to be a point where energy flows into the body and is associated with certain positive and negative qualities. For example, the throat chakra is linked to the thyroid gland and the body's metabolic rate. Thousands of 'energy channels', known as nadi, are said to cross the chakras and travel all over the body, carrying prana.

Practised regularly, yoga postures tone the body, maintain and increase suppleness, build stamina, improve the respiratory system, oxygenate the blood and keep the spine strong. Yoga is also said to sharpen the intellect and improve concentration, calm the mind and bring about inner peace.

Who uses yoga?

Today, in the West, yoga classes have sprung up everywhere: most health clubs run classes, as do adult education centres. There are also more and more centres dedicated almost entirely to teaching yoga and there are even some classes run in schools, offices, health centres and hospitals. Some people practise yoga to keep themselves healthy and fit, while others practise it because of a specific health problem such as back pain, stress, circulatory disorders, asthma, arthritis, digestive disorders or menstrual problems.

Is it effective?

In a survey published in *Which?* in December 2001, those practising yoga were the most satisfied with the therapy they were having, with

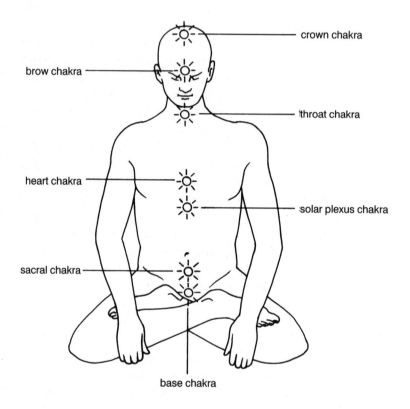

The major chakras

82 per cent of respondents saying they had been very satisfied with it, while 69 per cent said that it had greatly improved their specific health problem. Practised regularly, in the recommended way, the yoga postures stretch and tone nearly every muscle and tendon in the body and move nearly all the joints through their complete range of movement. There is no doubt that this stimulates the circulation and leads to an increase in suppleness and strength. Yoga also has an effect on the internal organs of the body, for example, doing a head stand improves blood flow to the brain, or doing twists gently massages the digestive system and liver and can help with the elimination of toxins and waste. It is important to practise a complete range of postures to get the full benefit: these include standing postures, forward bends, back bends, twists, balances and inverted postures. Whatever your ability at yoga, there will be postures in each group that you can do. The breathing techniques of yoga are also very beneficial, inducing relaxation, improving lung capacity and increasing energy.

There have been several studies on the benefits of yoga. Many uncontrolled observational studies have found yoga to have beneficial effects on mood, emotional well-being and quality of life in healthy people. A small number of controlled trials suggest that it can help for severe health problems, such as back problems, arthritis, diabetes, osteoporosis and high blood pressure. Yoga breathing has been shown to reduce the frequency of asthma attacks, and yoga meditation to benefit the heart and improve circulation.

A typical class

While you can learn yoga on your own, it is best to join a class to learn the basic techniques, then, if you like, you can practise at home. There are many different types of yoga (see below). Classes range from slow, meditative sessions through to dynamic and physically challenging forms of yoga; so, it is a good idea to go along and try a class out, to see if it is right for you and to make sure that you get on with the teacher. As yet, there is no regulatory body for standards of yoga teaching in the UK, so it is wise to ask for details of the teacher's training, qualifications and insurance. Also, there are different levels of yoga class, usually beginners, general and intermediate. If you have not done any yoga before, then you should start in a beginner's class. An intermediate class is usually only for people who have been practising for some years, as a good level of knowledge of the postures will be expected. A yoga session usually lasts 1–2 hours, depending on the type of yoga and level of the class.

Hatha yoga is concerned with the correct use (through exercise, breathing, relaxation, meditation and diet) of the complete body in order to bring the physical body into a perfect state of health, so that the 'soul' can be fully expressed through it. Today, it is the generic name given to the practice of yoga postures, breathing and relaxation. It is probably the name you are most likely to come across. Many of the other types of yoga are forms of hatha yoga.

Iyengar yoga was developed by BKS Iyengar, who still teaches at his Institute in Pune, India. A type of hatha yoga, Iyengar yoga calls the practice of asanas 'meditation in action' because it focuses the practitioner's attention on his or her own body and allows the senses to turn inwards in a similar way to sitting meditation. This form of yoga is now practised all over the world. Iyengar has systematically studied more than 200 yoga postures and breathing techniques and looked at how they relate to the anatomy of the body. From this he has found that, to get the best out of the postures and breathing, every part of the body needs to be positioned or aligned correctly. This type of yoga is characterised by precision and attention to detail in order to get the correct alignment in the yoga postures. It is quite a physically demanding system, but to enable everyone, whatever their ability, age or health status, to practise Iyengar yoga, various props such as blocks, chairs, belts and ropes are often used. This means it is also a good type of yoga to practise if you are ill or injured in any way, preferably under the guidance of an experienced Iyengar yoga teacher.

Astanga Vinyasa yoga, controversially also called 'Power yoga', was developed by K Pattabhi Jois, who learnt yoga from the same teacher as BKS Iyengar. The postures are similar to those practised in Iyengar yoga, but are carried out in set series. Usually, the postures are performed in a continuous flow, one after the other, often connected by jumps, and control of the breath is emphasised. This encourages a build-up of heat in the body. Less emphasis is put on the alignment of the body than in Iyengar yoga. It is a physically demanding system of yoga and you need to be relatively fit to attempt it.

Sivananda yoga is another form of hatha yoga, named after Swami Sivananda. It comprises a specific set of breathing practices and postures, and is probably less physically taxing than Astanga or Iyengar yoga, at least in the beginning.

Yoga therapy is a relatively new invention and is yoga specifically designed for people with a health problem. Yoga therapists are yoga teachers who have had additional training in how to use yoga to treat specific disorders.

Kundalini yoga comprises specific practices to raise the Kundalini energy that is said to reside in the base of the spine and to bring health, harmony and vitality when flowing well.

Tantric yoga is based on the belief that we can use the power of our senses and desires to transform and harmonise ourselves. It is the antithesis of the idea that we need to isolate ourselves from the world to reach enlightenment.

It is a good idea to practise yoga in a warm, draught-free room, on an empty stomach. It is best to wear unrestrictive clothing and to practise with bare feet; get a non-slip mat if your floor is slippery. The cost of a yoga class will vary from about £3–£15 depending on the location. An individual private lesson could cost anything from £50 per hour.

How safe is it?

Essentially, yoga is very safe and can be practised by young and old alike, whatever their level of fitness. However, there are some provisos. The postures need to be practised correctly, in the recommended sequence and at the right level for you. Forcing your body into an advanced position when it is not ready could lead to injury. It is always important to remember that yoga is not a competition to see who can get themselves into the most difficult posture. You may feel some muscle tenderness and joint stiffness after a yoga class, but you should never feel severe pain in a class or afterwards. Women should not perform inverted postures (for example, headstand and shoulder stand) when they are menstruating. There are also some people with certain diseases or injuries who need to take care with some of the postures and would benefit from careful supervision. A good teacher will check on his or her students' well-being and suggest suitable yoga practices to them. If you are concerned that yoga might be risky for you, talk to your doctor or a qualified yoga teacher about it. Yoga is not recommended during the first 14 weeks of pregnancy. Always tell your yoga teacher if you are pregnant, since pregnant women need to avoid certain postures at different times during their pregnancy. In fact, if you are pregnant and just starting to practise yoga, it is probably best to go to a special 'yoga for pregnancy' class.

Finding a yoga teacher

Yoga is a lifelong path – and so it is a good idea to go to a well-trained teacher. Those trained in the Iyengar system will have been practising Iyengar yoga intensively for a minimum of five years, including three years of training, just to be allowed to teach beginners' postures. It takes years of training and examinations before someone is allowed to teach advanced Iyengar postures or to teach remedial classes for people with a specific health problem. The British Wheel of Yoga★ also has a comprehensive training for its registered teachers, although it is less rigorous than that of the Iyengar system. Both the Iyengar Yoga Institute★ and the British Wheel regulate the standards of their own teachers and require that they are adequately insured to teach. The Yoga Biomedical Trust★ offers qualified yoga teachers a two-year training in yoga therapy for specific ailments.

Part III

Diagnostic techniques and other therapies

Diagnostic techniques

All of the main complementary systems of medicine, such as Traditional Chinese acupuncture and Ayurvedic medicine have their own diagnostic methods. There are also some complementary diagnostic techniques, such as radionics, iridology and Vega testing, which may be used by a range of different complementary practitioners; for example, naturopaths commonly use iridology to help them make a diagnosis.

Dowsing and radionic diagnosis

Radionics is a type of vibrational medicine, based on the belief that all life forms are connected to, and penetrated by, a common field of energy and that all matter emits radiation. It developed from the work and discoveries of an American doctor, Albert Abrams, in the early twentieth century and comprises absent diagnosis and absent healing (see page 104).

The aim of radionic diagnosis (radiesthesia) is to diagnose illness at a distance. This can involve using pendulums, hazel twigs, and quasi-scientific, electric instruments (not necessarily plugged in) to assess a person's energy, or measure the radiation he or she is emitting. It is not necessary to meet your radionics practitioner face to face; instead, you send him or her a sample from your body (usually hair, a nail clipping or a drop of blood) along with a completed medical questionnaire, from which the practitioner makes a diagnosis. These samples are known as the 'witness'. The practitioner puts the 'witness' into a 'black box'. This box is said to have frequency settings that are tuned to the vibrational levels of various diseases, rather like a radio. The practitioner uses these to try and pick up what is wrong with you from your samples. The box can also be used to send healing energy to the patient.

The practitioner may also dowse over the questionnaire and sample with a pendulum. The dowsing techniques used by practitioners of radionics are similar to those used in water divining. The latter involves walking over the ground carrying two metal rods or a forked, hazel twig, which dip when they cross a buried well or stream. A medical dowser uses a pendulum instead of a dowser's twig, and works from the 'witness' sent in by the patient. The pendulum, often a crystal on a chain, is held over the 'witness' and the practitioner observes whether it swings clockwise or anti-clockwise or to and fro. For each dowser, a certain movement of the pendulum means 'yes' and another 'no'. Dowsing is also used to select the 'correct' remedy for a patient, such as a herb or homeopathic remedy.

There have been no rigorous scientific tests of radionics or dowsing and many conventional healthcare practitioners and scientists are sceptical of it. By the same token, it is not considered to be harmful.

Finding a practitioner

The Radionics Association★ is the main organisation in the field, with its own School of Radionics. It takes about 18 months of part-time study to qualify as a licentiate of the Association and a further 18 months to qualify as a full member. Pupils who qualify are entitled to put MRadA (Member of the Radionic Association) after their name. A list of qualified members is available from the association for a small fee. A diagnosis costs about £25, then about £25 for subsequent monthly treatments. The British Society of Dowsers★ holds a series of short courses each year, has a Register of Practising Dowsers and offers a free public information service for those seeking the services of a dowser.

Hair analysis

Hair analysis is used predominantly by naturopaths and nutritional therapists, who believe that analysing strands of hair can indicate the levels of minerals in a person's body. The laboratory analysis of strands of hair has been used as a diagnostic technique since the nineteenth century.

The theory is that some of the chemicals we absorb into our bodies from food and the environment are stored in our hair. To maintain the correct workings of the body, these chemicals, such as essential minerals, are utilised and any excess is stored in body tissues such as the hair. Conversely, if we are not getting enough of these nutrients from our diets, a deficiency will show up in samples of our hair. Also, other chemicals, such as lead and mercury, which are toxic to the body and not vital to its function, are believed to accumulate in parts of the body such as the hair. Hair is made of keratin, a type of protein, and contains sulphur, which is said to trap minerals from the blood as it feeds the roots of the hair.

Hair analysis involves taking a 3cm sample of hair from the nape of your neck, near the root. This part of the hair contains the minerals that have been absorbed by your hair in the past three months. The sample is then sent to a laboratory, where it is burnt to an ash. It is this ash that is analysed for levels of essential minerals such as calcium, magnesium, phosphorus, potassium, sodium and toxic chemicals such as aluminium, arsenic, lead and mercury.

There is little scientific evidence to support the use of hair analysis to diagnose disease. While it may be able to tell something about your long-term exposure to toxic chemicals from a sample of your hair, hair analysis is not thought to be a reliable way of measuring the mineral content of the body or making other diagnoses.

Finding a practitioner

The sections on naturopathy and nutritional therapy explain how to find a qualified naturopath or nutritional therapist.

Iridology

Iridology is a diagnostic technique that involves studying the irises of the eyes (the coloured part) for abnormalities, such as character-istic markings and colour. It is based on the belief that each area of the body and all the organs are mapped on specific parts of the iris, the right iris corresponding to organs on the right-hand side of the body and the left iris to those on the left side. The version we know today was developed by a Hungarian physician, Ignatz von Peczely, over 100 years ago, although there are stone slabs with carvings of the iris on them that date back to 1000BC. Iridology is now popular with naturopaths and many other complementary therapists.

The iridology maps that Peczely first developed have since been refined, and today practitioners claim that the charts (see page 178) enable them to detect past, present and future physical and psychological problems because the iris provides a blueprint of a person's genetic and constitutional strengths and weaknesses. However, iridologists do not claim to be able to diagnose specific diseases but maintain that they can identify physical weakness that could lead to disease. So, for example, an abnormality on the part of the iris that corresponds to the heart is said to indicate a weakness with the heart itself. Iridologists examine the eye using a torch and a magnifying glass, then make notes of what they see. Some also use a special camera to film the eyes so that the patient can also see what is going on. They claim that a healthy iris is clear and uniform, whatever the colour.

Most conventional healthcare professionals are not impressed with the evidence for iridology and ophthalmologists do not recognise iridology as having any place in medicine. Sparkly, bright eyes are usually taken as a sign of good health, and certain specific changes indicate specific illnesses, such as a milky ring surrounding the iris, which is an indication of hardening of the arteries due to high cholesterol, or a yellow tinge to the whites of the eyes, which is a sign of jaundice. However, there is little convincing research to show that the body is mapped out on the irises or that iridology can diagnose disease. While iridologists claim that the thousands of nerve endings in the iris link it to every body organ and tissue, there are no known neural connections between the iris and other organs of the body to explain iridology. Furthermore, a systematic review of four controlled trials of iridology found that the method is no more likely to diagnose a specific weakness than chance.

If an iridologist feels that you could have a serious disease, you should be advised to see a GP, especially if the practitioner subscribes to a professional code of ethics. However, some ophthalmologists report that they have examined patients who have been diagnosed incorrectly by iridologists, and whose irises were normal. The iris cannot develop new markings overnight; nor does it change colour, except under certain rare circumstances, such as a severe retinal problem. In all, it is dangerous to rely on iridology for a diagnosis. If you feel ill, see a doctor, not an iridologist.

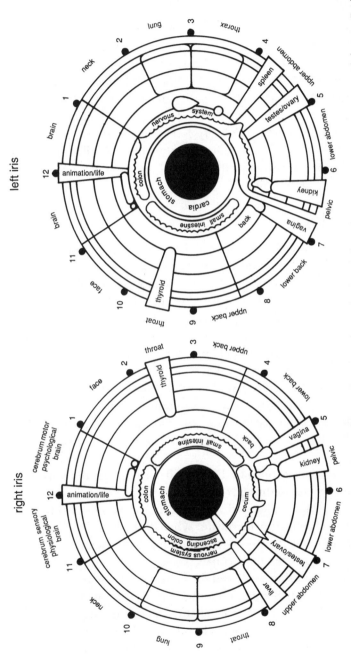

Each iris is divided into 12 radial sections, which correspond to an area of the body, such as lower abdomen, face or upper abdomen. Each section is further sub-divided so that areas within one section could cover the kidneys, adrenal glands, scrotum and so on. In addition, the map is divided into circular zones that indicate different tissues and body systems, such as arteries and blood, muscle or skin.

Finding a practitioner

Anybody can set him- or herself up as an iridologist; it is a completely unregulated technique. There are about 300 qualified iridologists in the UK, who are registered with one of two organisations that each has its own code of conduct and ethics: the Guild of Naturopathic Iridologists★, which is affiliated to the Institute for Complementary Medicine (ICM)★, and the International Association of Clinical Iridologists★. The first session of iridology, which lasts about an hour, will cost about £30–£50, depending on your location, and about half that for shorter follow-up sessions. Often one session is enough.

Kinesiology

Kinesiology, also known as applied kinesiology, comprises a complementary diagnostic technique and also sometimes treatment. It was developed by a US chiropractor called George Goodheart in the 1960s. It is based on the beliefs that our bodies 'know' why we are ill or in pain, and that ill health can be caused by the accumulation of toxins around major muscle groups in the body, such as the biceps in the upper arms or the quadriceps in the thigh. This then leads to weakness in the specific muscle groups around which the toxins have built up. Kinesiologists believe that the relative strengths or weaknesses of different muscle groups can be used to determine a person's health, and allergies or food intolerances, because certain muscle groups correspond to certain body systems.

The theory developed by Dr Goodheart was that the muscles, organs and glands of the body are connected by a network of energy pathways, which include the nerves, blood vessels, lymphatic system and acupuncture meridians. When the body is out of balance owing to illness, an 'overload' of toxins, injury or stress, the energy circuit to certain muscles becomes blocked or 'switched off'. This muscle then becomes weak, and the corresponding body system or systems stop functioning properly, which can then result in symptoms. Kinesiologists test the strength of the various muscle groups to see which ones are weak and which body systems are out of balance. One of the main uses of kinesiology today is to test for allergies and food intolerances. To do this, the kinesiologist will place a nutrient or chemical directly on to your tongue or skin, or in a phial placed on your body, to 'stimulate' your energy pathways. If you are allergic or intolerant to the substance under test, it will trigger your muscles to turn on or off. The kinesiologist will use one of your major muscle groups, such as your biceps, to test your reaction to the substance. If the muscles sag or feel weak, this is said to indicate that you are allergic or intolerant to it or perhaps that you have accumulated it in your body. Conversely, if your muscles strengthen this is said to indicate that you are deficient in that substance and will benefit from it.

There is no existing scientific rationale for how kinesiology might work. Also, it has been assessed in several rigorous randomised controlled trials, which have all shown that it is no more likely than chance to be able to diagnose a disease or allergy. As well as using kinesiology as a diagnostic technique, kinesiologists use a range of treatments which, they claim, restore energy flow and muscle balance. These include manipulation to improve nerve and blood supply; massage and touch to stimulate blood circulation and to balance emotions; and nutritional support and advice. They maintain that their techniques can help with many niggling emotional and physical problems that may lead to illness.

Finding a practitioner

Kinesiology is currently unregulated: there are about 600 kinesiologists in the UK and about 16 schools of kinesiology. The latter include polarity reflex analysis, biokinesiology, systematic kinesiology/ balanced health and touch for health, but the principles of all of these are essentially the same. The Kinesiology Federation★ is an umbrella organisation that covers most of these schools and has a membership of about 300 practising kinesiologists. The minimum requirements for membership are 150 hours of training and 200 hours of clinical experience within a period of two to three years. The Federation has codes of conduct and ethics, and a disciplinary procedure; its members must be insured. The other main organisation is the Association of Systematic Kinesiology★, which has about 135 individual members. Its training takes 40 days, spread over two to three years. Kinesiology is also used as a diagnostic technique by chiropractors, nutritionists, osteopaths and even some conventional practitioners. An initial kinesiology session takes about an hour and can cost from £20–£50; subsequent visits cost about £15–£35. Usually, you will need between one and six sessions.

Kirlian photography

Kirlian photography is a technique used to photograph the electro-magnetic energy field (known as the bioenergetic corona discharge) around any living tissue. In the case of humans, and probably other living beings, this is said to change shape and colour according to our emotional state, vitality and health. Some practitioners interpret the field as the aura (see Glossary) that healers claim to be able to see around people.

Kirlian photography involves placing the subject to be photographed in a high-frequency alternating electric field. This field is said to interact with the energy field around the subject being photographed and the resulting 'interference pattern' is manifested on to a photographic plate. A Russian husband and wife team (Semyon and Valentina Kirlian) developed the technique. While they were repairing an electrotherapy machine that was used to treat paralysis, Semyon noticed a weak luminous glow between his hand and the part of the machine responsible for conducting electricity. When they photographed the phenomenon on to light-sensitive paper, it showed up as streams of light coming from his fingertips.

Today, if you undergo a Kirlian photographic diagnosis, you will be asked to place your hand (or sometimes foot) for one minute on photographic paper placed on top of an aluminium plate protected by glass. This plate is then linked to a power unit known as a Tesla coil. While an electric charge is running through the plate, you will feel a tingling sensation in your hand. The resulting photograph is usually developed immediately and a diagnosis is made based on comparisons with other Kirlian photographs and the practitioner's own intuition. The practitioner may then refer you to a doctor or another complementary therapist, depending on the diagnosis.

While Kirlian photography has been shown in some – but not all – studies to be better than chance at diagnosing disease, it is less sensitive than conventional medical diagnostic tests. Also, the tech-nique does not appear to be repeatable between various investi-gators and it has not been possible to use the technique in routine diagnosis. Kirlian photography has been used to photograph acupuncture points, and the hands of healers during healing sessions, which are said to give off a flare visible on the photographs. What is actually being photographed has not been explained scientifically and sceptics say that a person's body temperature, and the voltage and frequency of the electrical charge used, can all distort the patterns created and may even account for them.

Finding a practitioner

Very few complementary therapists use Kirlian photography.

Reflexology maps

The reflexology charts (see pages 152–3) used by reflexologists are sometimes used to make a diagnosis of what is wrong with you, as well as being used as a basis for reflexology treatment. As explained in the section on reflexology, the charts consist of pictures of the soles and the tops of the feet, on which the corresponding organs or parts of the body are superimposed.

Reputable reflexology organisations now insist that their members do not use reflexology as a diagnostic tool because it could lead to unnecessary medical treatment or worse, no treatment, when such would be vital. However, an underpinning theory in reflexology is that when a certain part of the body is diseased or 'out of balance', the corresponding part of the foot will be tender and feel 'gritty'. Reflexologists use this to guide their treatments; if a reflexologist suspects from an assessment of your feet that there may be a serious underlying condition, he or she should advise you to see your GP.

The results of scientific investigations of the value of reflexology charts to diagnose disease have been inconsistent. Studies have found that reflexologists are no more likely than chance to be able to make an accurate diagnosis. One study found that blood flow through the kidneys increased when the corresponding reflexology zone on the foot was massaged.

Finding a practitioner

For information about how to find a reflexologist, see the section on reflexology.

Vega testing

Vega testing is a diagnostic technique based on measuring abnormalities in the electrical properties of acupuncture points. It was developed by a German doctor, Reinhold Voll, in the 1950s, after he discovered that acupuncture points had electrical properties. During his research, Dr Voll also claimed to find new points that related to specific organs in the body.

About 20 years later, another German doctor, Helmut Schimmel, designed a simple machine known as a vega machine, based on Dr Voll's work. Still used today, the vega machine measures the electrical properties of acupuncture points. A vega test involves connecting you to an electrical device to test your reaction to different homeopathic dilutions of various substances, such as suspected allergens (substances that trigger an allergic reaction in you), bacteria and viruses that you might be infected with, and diseased tissue. The theory is that if you react to a substance this will show up as a disturbance on the vega machine. Different practitioners have different theories as to why such a disturbance occurs. Some explain it using the theories of Traditional Chinese Medicine (TCM) and claim that the machine measures changes in Qi flowing through the meridians of the body, while others believe that body cells vibrate at different frequencies and the machine measures changes in these frequencies. During a test, a low voltage current is applied via an electronic probe to certain acupuncture points on your hands, feet and possibly your head that are said to correspond with different organs. Then, the homeopathic dilutions are linked into the electrical circuit. Any changes in the readings on the machine induced by one of these substances are believed to indicate that you have a sensitivity to the substance and are either allergic to it or ill because of it. Practitioners who use vega testing claim that it can also be used to identify what substances you should be treated with.

There is no scientific rationale for vega testing, and little evidence to indicate that it is a valid diagnostic technique. Most trials testing the accuracy of the technique have found it to be no more accurate than chance at diagnosing illness. They have also found that results obtained with vega testing are not reproducible. In one trial, vega testing was successful in identifying people with health problems most of the time, but could not actually diagnose what types of disease they had.

Finding a practitioner

A significant number of complementary therapists from a variety of disciplines, such as homeopaths and acupuncturists, use Vega testing. To find a qualified practitioner, see the appropriate section in Part II of this book.

Other therapies in brief

This section gives a brief overview of most of the other complementary therapies and practices available in the UK. These therapies tend to be less widely available and less well accepted by conventional healthcare practitioners than those discussed in Part II. Generally, there has been less scientific research investigating these therapies and little is known about their effectiveness. This does not mean that they do not work, just that we do not yet have the scientific evidence to show that they do.

Anthroposophical medicine

Anthroposophical medicine forms part of Rudolf Steiner's philosophy of anthroposophy. It embodies a holistic approach to health and medicine that integrates conventional approaches with complementary therapies and an exploration of inner feelings and the meaning of illness.

Rudolf Steiner (1861–1925) was an Austrian scientist and philosopher who founded a new kind of science in which both the human being and the natural world are described in terms of the soul and spirit, as well as the physical. He developed it because he believed that the reductionist approach of modern science, in which all phenomena are reduced to physical events, cannot explain the experience of life, feeling and consciousness. He did not see his approach as an alternative to science but as an extension of it. It was only in his later years that Steiner concerned himself with the field of medicine and worked with doctors who believed that anthroposophy could make a valuable contribution to medicine.

Anthroposophical medicine is based on the concept that there are four distinct aspects to the human being: the 'physical' body, the 'etheric' body (similar to Qi in acupuncture or prana in Ayurveda), the 'astral' body (the soul) and the 'ego' (the human intelligent self). These four aspects are inter-related and good health depends on a harmonious relationship between them, and an imbalance in one body can cause disturbances in the other three. The anthroposophical doctor seeks to understand illness in a person in terms of this inter-relation. Also, in a similar way to naturopathy, life is deemed to depend on the dynamic balance between catabolism (the breaking down and using of energy) and anabolism (the building up and storing of energy). This concept is known as Steiner's 'principle of polarity'. Anatomically, it corresponds to the nerves (catabolism) and blood (anabolism), while physiologically, it corresponds to waking (catabolism) and sleeping (anabolism). The two poles are said to be linked and harmonised by a rhythmic system comprising the chest (that is, the heart, lungs, and circulatory and respiratory systems as a whole). This view of the human being is very different from the conventional view that all functions of the mind and soul are centred in the brain, as it implies that our feelings and emotions are centred in the rhythmic system. The aim of anthroposophical medicine is to stimulate the natural healing forces within the human being.

Anthroposophical medicine can be used to treat any illness. However, little specific scientific research has been carried out to assess the effectiveness of anthroposophical medicine. One uncontrolled study at the Royal London Homeopathic Hospital found that anthroposophically based cancer care, which included the anthroposophical medicine Iscador (an extract of mistletoe), enhanced the patients' quality of life. There are no specific safety concerns with anthroposophical medicine, but the safety concerns of any individual therapy used within its context obviously apply.

Finding a practitioner

Currently, anthroposophical medicine is most widely used in Germany, the Netherlands and Switzerland, where there are two general hospitals in which it is integrated with modern medicine and eight specialised anthroposophical hospitals, as well as hundreds of general practitioners and specialists who use it. In the UK, relatively few practitioners and services provide this type of medicine, although there are several Steiner schools, some of which cater for children with special needs, and a residential therapeutic centre that provides anthroposophical medical treatment.

Practitioners are fully qualified doctors. A consultation with an anthroposophical doctor takes up to an hour, during which time you will be asked questions about your health, lifestyle, diet and constitution. The doctor will also take a conventional medical history, carry out a physical examination and may order laboratory tests and radiographic investigations. Usually, you will be prescribed anthroposophical medicines, which are made from plants, animals and minerals and are prepared in the same way as homeopathic remedies, along with conventional medicines. Other therapies might include massage, hydrotherapy, eurythmy (a movement therapy developed by Steiner), art therapies and special diets. A list of anthroposophical practitioners can be obtained from the Anthroposophical Medical Association★. The length of treatment and number of consultations vary from individual to individual, as does the cost of the treatment. There are a few anthroposophical NHS GPs. Patients on their lists receive free advice and those medicines available on the NHS via an NHS prescription; patients not on their lists will be expected to pay a modest fee.

Art therapy

Art therapy is the use of creative art as a means of expression for rehabilitation and personal development. In the UK, art therapy was developed in the 1940s when the artist, Adrian Hill, began to work informally with patients in sanatoriums and when artists, keen to work with the sick and wounded, were employed in hospitals and clinics to work with rehabilitating soldiers during the Second World War. In Europe, Rudolf Steiner (see page 185) included art therapy as part of anthroposophical medicine and both Freud and Jung, in the early 1920s, believed that visual images could reflect a patient's subconscious state. Today, art therapy is used by doctors, psychiatrists and psychotherapists worldwide to help people with physical, mental, emotional or learning problems.

Art therapy is a form of self-exploration and works by allowing people to express their feelings through painting, sculpting, modelling, collage and drawing. At the first session, the art therapist will make an assessment about your condition and ask about your life situation and any emotional problems you have. In a session, you are offered crayons, charcoal, clay and Plasticine as well as paper, cardboard, fabric and old newspapers and can use the materials in any way you wish to express your thoughts and feelings. You do not have to be artistic to gain benefit from art therapy. The art form is a means to an end, to take you out of yourself and allow you to express emotions, such as anger and grief, which are hard to put into words. Once you have created your art form, you will then work with the art therapist, either separately or in a group, to explore the meaning of what you have created. Over a period of time, art therapy can help a person learn all sorts of things about his or her life and personality, which may previously have been 'hidden'.

There are different ways of working within art therapy. Some art therapists do not directly interpret a person's work, particularly those coming from a traditional art therapy background (started by artists who worked in hospitals). This type of art therapist believes that it is the individual who holds the key to the interpretation of his or her work, and that the individual and his or her artwork is central to the process. However, art therapists from a psychotherapy background believe that a more directed approach is needed, within which the art is used as a non-verbal therapeutic dialogue between the patient and the therapist. In this type of art therapy – sometimes referred to as art psychotherapy – the therapeutic relationship, rather than the artwork, is central to the process.

Art therapy is said to benefit people who are suffering from drug or alcohol problems, eating disorders, mental and emotional disorders such as psychosis, depression and anxiety, learning difficulties, bereavement, stress, dementia or a terminal illness. It is also used as a personal development tool and to help those who have difficulty in expressing their feelings. For example, older people can find art therapy a good way of expressing their emotions when they are having to cope with experiences such as losing their home and moving into institutional care. It is also used in other institutions, such as prisons and rehabilitation centres.

There is little scientific evidence in support of art therapy from well-controlled clinical trials but a wealth of case studies, from both Europe and North America, has shown the value of art therapy for a wide range of problems, including severe learning difficulties, eating disorders, alcohol and drug addictions, and psychotic illness.

Finding a practitioner

The British Association of Art Therapists* was established in 1963 and now lists about 1,000 practitioners. Since 1997, art therapy has been a state-registered therapy and is classified as a profession allied to medicine, which means it is illegal for unqualified practitioners to call themselves an art therapist. Qualified art therapists can be recognised by the initials RATh (Registered Art Therapist). Therapists must be graduates, usually in art, and have completed a postgraduate Diploma of Art Therapy, which takes three or four years of full-time training and involves developing one's own artistic skills – and a recognition of how these are interconnected with inner development and an understanding of the whole human being – as well as practical placements. Art therapy has been recognised by the NHS since 1982 and therapists often work in a hospital or clinical setting in the areas of physical or mental illness, disabilities or learning difficulties. Some therapists also work from their own studios, where a private session costs around £30–£40, but most of their clients are referred to them from teachers or doctors.

Bowen technique

The Bowen technique was developed by an Australian bodyworker, Tom Bowen, in the 1950s. It involves gently moving soft tissue such as muscles and tendons using pressure from the thumbs and fingers. Its aim is to stimulate energy flow in the body, so stimulating the self-healing capabilities within the body and restoring normal structure. It is used to treat muscle and joint problems, back pain, sports injuries, stress-related disorders and symptoms of chronic conditions.

Bowen moves are a form of gentle but precise soft tissue manipulation. The therapist makes light, rolling movements with his or her thumbs or fingers. This is believed to encourage circulation of blood and lymph, and increase mobility, and is also said to release blocked energy. The Bowen technique is very gentle and subtle; the therapist does not seek to force or directly realign the body to fit a preconceived form or state of health. Neither do Bowen therapists attempt to make a diagnosis. They claim to be holistic, focusing on the whole patient throughout the treatment and with no rigid idea of how your body will receive the moves and use them. They believe that all human bodies are different and each body will have its own interpretation of disease and injury, and its own response, either to a named disease or injury or a specific treatment.

At a first session, the Bowen therapist will make a note of your medical history, although few of the Bowen moves are intended to resolve a particular problem. The therapy is carried out on a low, soft treatment table. You will not be asked to undress but to wear loose, comfortable clothing. If you are planning to have Bowen therapy, you will be asked not to have any other physical therapy in the five days prior to receiving it and for two weeks afterwards. The reason given for this is because to do so would overload you with messages that, in turn, would neutralise the 'subtle power' of the Bowen treatment. A unique feature of the Bowen technique is that there are frequent breaks in a treatment session in which the therapist leaves not just the patient but the treatment room. These breaks are believed to be essential, as they enable the body to absorb the information presented by the therapist and to allow the body time for healing processes to begin. Furthermore, these breaks are seen to play an important role in ensuring that the healing of the patient is not overly dependent upon the presence of the therapist. On returning, the therapist will note changes in muscle tension or body alignment or comments made by the patient. The subsequent Bowen moves that the therapist makes will be determined more by this new information than by a preordained sequence of moves. Bowen therapists also believe that the effectiveness of a treatment can be reduced, if more information is presented to the body than it can deal with. The therapist may therefore decide to end the session at an earlier moment than anticipated. The therapist may also give you a programme of exercises. Flower essences, homeopathy or herbal medicine can be used in conjunction with Bowen.

The most frequent immediate response to Bowen treatment is a deep sense of relaxation and well-being. There is little scientific evidence to support the theories underpinning the Bowen technique or to support its effectiveness. There are no known safety concerns with this technique, but occasionally people report feeling a little unsettled, or even dizzy, after a treatment.

Finding a practitioner

The Bowen technique is completely unregulated. To find a practitioner trained in the Bowen technique contact the Bowen Therapists

European Register (BTER)★, which is the largest Bowen therapist organisation in Europe. All therapists on its register must have a qualification in the Bowen technique, anatomy and physiology (or equivalent other therapy), a current first aid certificate, professional indemnity insurance and have undertaken additional Bowen studies of at least 14 hours in the previous year. Each session of the Bowen technique lasts about 30–40 minutes and the average course of treatments is two to three sessions. For prices contact the individual practitioners.

Chelation therapy

Chelation therapy is used in an 'alternative' way to treat arterial diseases such as coronary heart disease and stroke by more than 1,000 physicians in the USA. In the UK, however, its use in this way is controversial, although it is an established conventional treatment for heavy metal poisoning.

In conventional medicine, chelation therapy involves giving a synthetic form of the amino acid EDTA (ethylene diamine tetra-acetic acid) to chemically remove, or chelate, heavy metals such as lead and cadmium from the bloodstream – such heavy metals are known to be very toxic to the body. Apparently, its complementary use developed after some doctors noticed that other conditions, such as heart disease and peripheral arterial disease, also improved in some patients treated with chelation therapy.

Chelation therapy must be carried out under the supervision of a qualified doctor. At a first session, the doctor will normally take a conventional medical history and make a conventional diagnosis. Treatment involves inserting an intravenous drip into your arm containing a solution of EDTA, heparin, vitamins and minerals. The doctor will also need to monitor your circulation, blood pressure, cholesterol and blood sugar levels, and kidney and other organ function throughout the treatment.

The main complementary uses for chelation therapy are in heart disease, peripheral vascular disease, and stroke prevention, or as an alternative to coronary artery bypass graft surgery. It has also been claimed to help in arthritis, impaired vision, hearing or memory, diabetes, high blood pressure, osteoporosis, Parkinson's disease, kidney disease and gallstones. Although there has been research in to the use of chelation therapy as a treatment for heart and circulatory diseases, there is little good evidence to support its use in the treatment of these or any other conditions. Anecdotal data suggest that up to 80 per cent of people benefit, but a systematic review of four randomised, double-blind, placebo-controlled trials assessing the effectiveness of chelation therapy for peripheral artery disease found the evidence to be unconvincing, while another systematic review of clinical studies of chelation therapy for heart disease concluded that the treatment should now be considered obsolete. The quality of these trials has been called into question. Chelation therapy should not be used during pregnancy nor in people with kidney problems or bleeding abnormalities. It can cause unwanted effects such as kidney failure, abnormal heartbeats, low blood sugar, low blood pressure and seizures.

Finding a practitioner

A number of NHS health authorities have funded a few patients to have chelation therapy privately, while a similar number have refused NHS funding. The Department of Health is awaiting the results of large-scale clinical trials before it endorses chelation therapy for arterial disease. To find a doctor who uses chelation therapy in an alternative way, contact the Arterial Disease Foundation★. A treatment can last from about 1–3 hours and a course of treatments often involves having 10–30 sessions in total over the course of several months. For costs contact the individual practitioners.

Colonic irrigation

Colonic irrigation or *lavage*, also known as colonic hydrotherapy or colon therapy, is a complementary technique that is used for bowel problems such as constipation and irritable bowel syndrome and is also used as a detoxification process. Records of colonic irrigation and enemas date back over 4,000 years to Egyptian artefacts, but colonic irrigation as we know it today dates back to the mid nineteenth century and the advent of spa therapy, and to the use of enemas in conventional medicine to ensure daily bowel movements. Today, in conventional medicine, the use of enemas has been replaced in favour of the use of powerful laxatives, as these are quicker and easier to administer. However, colonic irrigation is still advocated by many naturopaths and some other complementary practitioners, particularly as a means of detoxifying the body with the aim of treating a wide range of conditions including allergies and addictions.

Colonic irrigation involves introducing water, sometimes with coffee, herbs or enzymes added, into the colon to flush it out. The difference between an enema and colonic irrigation is that in the former the tube is not inserted very far up into the colon and water is retained in the bowel and expelled in the toilet, while in the latter, more fluid is pumped into the patient, through the whole length of the large intestine, and a constant flow of liquid in and out washes the whole colon. The theory behind colonic irrigation is that an 'unhealthy' colon is one that has become clogged up with impacted faecal matter, gases and mucus deposits, which proliferate due to the Western diet because of the many refined food products it contains. All this matter, therapists claim, becomes trapped in folds in the colon wall, leading to a build-up of toxins, which inhibits the natural movement of the gut and leads to constipation and compromised elimination processes. Flushing out the colon is also said to remove 'harmful' bacteria and give 'good' bacteria, such as *lactobacilli*, a better chance to proliferate.

On your first visit for colonic irrigation, the practitioner will take a full case history and explain the procedure. He or she will usually be trained in another complementary therapy, such as naturopathy, and will almost invariably give you advice on your diet and lifestyle. You will be asked to lie on your side on a table, wearing a gown, and the therapist will gently insert a lubricated sterilised speculum a few centimetres into your anus. You will then have to lie on your back with your knees bent up while water is gently pumped into the lower 1.5m of the intestine via a sterile tube, at a low pressure. The tube in your rectum is attached to two smaller tubes at the base (like an inverted Y). Through one of these tubes warm water is pumped into the large intestine and through the other waste matter is drained away. The outlet tube is transparent, so the therapist can see the nature of the waste passed during treatment. The therapist then lightly massages the stomach to stimulate the release of matter. The temperature of the water may be adjusted during the treatment to influence the muscles of your bowel. Warmer water relaxes them and slows the movement of your bowel, while cooler water stimulates bowel action. A session takes about 30–45 minutes. At the end of it you are told to visit the lavatory to get rid of any remaining water and then given a *Lactobacillus acidophilus* drink to 'restore' your 'good' gut flora.

Claims have been made that occasional but regular colonic irrigation clears the skin, prevents headaches, improves circulation, helps in the reduction of weight, alleviates the symptoms of chronic fatigue syndrome and relieves depression. It is also said to relieve the symptoms of irritable bowel syndrome, particularly if it is used in conjunction with herbal, dietary or homeopathic treatment. However, there is little scientific evidence to support the use of colonic irrigation, and the idea that our digestive systems are full of toxins and bacteria, which have to be flushed away to achieve good health, is dismissed as nonsense by gastroenterologists. The colon is naturally populated by a variety of bacteria, the main function of which is to break down fibre. Not only are these bacteria vital for digestion, but they appear to have a beneficial effect on the lining of the digestive tract. Flushing out waste matter removes the material on which the bacteria feed and can upset the delicate balance of our intestines. Drinking a glass of *Lactobacillus acidophilus* after flushing out the colon will make little or no difference.

People who have experienced colonic irrigation say that the procedure is not uncomfortable. Most claim to feel light-headed and elated afterwards. There are risks with colonic irrigation including infections, perforation of the colon if the pressure of the water pumped into the bowel is too high, and electrolyte imbalance caused by depriving the body of salt, water and potassium. There have even been some deaths associated with the procedure. Colonic irrigation should not be carried out during pregnancy, or in someone with high blood pressure or active inflammatory bowel disease or an acute infectious disease.

Finding a practitioner

If you feel you must have colonic irrigation, make sure that the therapist is a member of the Association and Register of Colon Hydrotherapists★. To remain a member of the organisation, the practitioner is required to attend a two-day seminar every year and have his or her premises inspected annually. The cost of one session of colonic irrigation is between £30 and £60, depending on your location. An initial course usually comprises six sessions, at weekly or fortnightly intervals, and a one-off 'spring-clean' every six months is often recommended.

Colour therapy

Colour therapy involves shining single or mixed colours on the whole body or on to particular areas, such as the chakras. Many ancient civilisations, including the Egyptians, Greeks and Chinese, used the healing properties of colours to restore health and vitality in their patients: the walls of Egyptian and Greek healing temples, for example, were painted in colours that were thought to be significant and very deliberately chosen. In ancient China, people suffering from chickenpox were wrapped in red silk and put out in the sun, which is said to have prevented scarring. Dinshah Ghadiali, an Indian scientist, made the first attempt at a scientific explanation of colour therapy, in the early twentieth century. Today, colour therapists believe that different colours can treat physical and mental health and improve the mind, body and spirit.

Moods have long been associated with colour, our language even reflects this: we are 'green' with envy or jealousy, 'blue' when we are down, 'see red' when we are angry and become 'white' or 'purple' with rage. Moreover, interior designers and psychologists claim that the colour of a room has an effect on people sitting in the room: for instance, blue is considered soothing, green calming and yellow warming. Colour therapy takes this one step further. It is based on the theory that the vibrations of colour waves have a direct effect on the cells and organs of our bodies. Because each colour has a specific wavelength and frequency, every colour is said to have its own unique vibration. Colour therapists also believe that our cells and organs vibrate at certain frequencies and that they can use colours to correct vibrational imbalances in the body, so creating balance, and good health and well-being. Each colour is thought to have different and specific effects on the body.

Some practitioners also submit to the theory that the human body has an aura around it made up of different colours that reflects our physical, emotional and spiritual health, and that our bodies absorb light waves and emit them in the form of an aura. According to colour therapists, if we become emotionally or mentally upset, a change in the auric colours results, which alters the vibrational frequency of the physical body. If this is not rectified, it will eventually manifest itself as a physical disease. Some practitioners claim that they can 'see' a person's aura. Many colour therapists also use the Ayurvedic theory of the body's chakras (see page 165). Light is thought to stream into the body through the chakras, each of which corresponds to a particular colour, part of the body and certain emotions. The chakra at the crown corresponds to the colour magenta, at the forehead – violet, the throat – blue, the heart – green, the solar plexus – yellow, the lower abdomen – orange and the base of the coccyx – red.

The first session with a colour therapist takes about two hours. The therapist will ask you about your health and whether you are taking any medication, and will then decide what colours should be 'applied'. Those therapists who claim to be able to 'see' auras will use this to guide them in choosing the most appropriate colour, or colours, for you. Others may ask you to choose a colour from a range of cards or bottles filled with coloured liquid, believing that the colour you choose reveals important traits of your personality. Some colour therapists dowse (see page 173) a colour chart to establish what colours you need. Colour therapy sets out to alleviate the effects of disease by immersing a part of the body or the whole body in a particular colour or colours. Different conditions are believed to respond to different colours: for example, blue is used to treat insomnia or high blood pressure, magenta for compulsive behaviour, violet to treat addictions, green for nervous tension, yellow for arthritis, orange to lift depression, red to treat inertia and turquoise (for which there is no corresponding chakra) to strengthen the immune system. The main colour chosen is usually given with a complementary colour (for example, green with magenta), to enhance the former's power. Colour can be applied in a number of ways – through stained-glass filters either to the whole body or to a part of the body, or by laying crystals on the person. Other colour therapy tools include silk scarves, clothing and coloured water. Your colour therapist may also advise you to wear certain colours, and include them in your diet and environment and may even teach you how to visualise (see page 226) yourself breathing in a certain colour or bathing in its light.

Colour therapists do not claim to be able cure you, but say they can improve a person's health and that, if an illness is treated early enough, it is possible to reverse the process of the illness. There is no scientific evidence for vibrational healing through colour, or for auras or chakras; however, there is considerable evidence to show that colour can affect mood. For example, one study showed that yellow could increase learning ability in children, while another showed that yellow, orange or red in the classroom increased the students' IQ. Other studies have found that blue is a calming colour and can slow heart rate and lower blood pressure, while red is stimulating and can increase heart rate and cause blood pressure to rise. There are few risks with colour therapy, as long as people are aware that it does not offer a cure. People suffering from high blood pressure, epilepsy, heart disease and asthma should not be subjected to red light, while those suffering from depression should not be given blue light, as this can aggravate the condition.

Finding a practitioner

Colour therapy is unregulated. There are around 600 colour therapists in the UK but some have no training and may charge substantial sums of money for sitting you under a series of randomly changing lights. The umbrella organisation for colour therapy is the International Association of Colour Therapy★. A person who wishes to obtain a basic certificate in colour therapy has to undertake a year's part-time course of academic and clinical work; for a diploma, a practitioner must submit a thesis of 25,000–35,000 words. The initials to look out for after a practitioner's name are HCertCTh (Hygeia Certificate of Colour Therapy), HDipCTh (Hygeia Diploma of Colour Therapy) and IACT (International Association for Colour Therapy). After working for two years, a colour therapist can apply for membership of the Institute for Complementary Medicine (ICM)★. The first session of colour therapy lasts about an hour and will cost around £45; subsequent sessions cost about £25 and are slightly shorter. The number of sessions required will depend on whether you have an acute or chronic problem.

Crystal healing

Crystal healing, or crystal therapy, is the use of crystals to influence the body's 'energy field' or aura in order to bring about healing and harmony. The belief that crystals (precious and semi-precious gems such as diamonds, rubies and emeralds are all crystals) have magical and healing properties has a long history. Many spiritual healers now use crystals to help with a wide range of physical and emotional conditions.

Crystal therapists believe that crystals can tap into the 'energies of the universe', focus 'healing energy' and resonate with the 'energies of the body' to bring about healing. Crystals are individually selected for their energy. Crystals such as amethyst and rose quartz are particularly thought to possess healing energy, which they can store and release rather like a battery. Practitioners claim that the crystals do not actually heal a person but rather act as a focus to help people heal themselves.

You can either buy your own crystals or visit a therapist. If you choose to do the latter, on your first visit you may be questioned about your lifestyle, diet and medical history, then asked to sit or lie on a couch or the floor. You will not need to undress. The therapist will then use his or her intuition to scan your energy, without actually touching you, or dowse (see page 173) or muscle test (see page 177), to assess which crystals to use. He or she may place crystals around you or on the part of your body that needs healing, may hold them him- or herself, ask you to hold them, or may use a combination of these approaches. Some practitioners place the crystals on acupuncture points or chakras; others combine crystal healing with spiritual healing and aura work. The skill of the practitioner is in choosing which crystal to use and applying it in the most effective way for the person being treated.

Crystal therapists do not claim to treat specific conditions, saying that they take a holistic approach and that crystal healing creates general good health and well-being. Anecdotally, some people report that they find that holding, wearing, being covered in or surrounded by crystals makes them feel better and more 'energised'. Some research has shown that if a quartz crystal is held in the hand for more than 30 minutes, brainwave patterns change from beta (fully alert) to alpha (relaxed). However, there is no scientific evidence to show that crystals have healing properties. There are no known safety concerns, as long as you consult a doctor if you feel unwell.

Finding a practitioner

The Affiliation of Crystal Healing Organisations* was set up in 1988 to act as a representative body for 12 crystal healing organisations. All the registered practitioners undergo a minimum of two years' part-time training, are insured and are obliged to adhere to a code of conduct. A session of crystal healing lasts between 40 and 90 minutes and will cost you between £10 and £30 depending on your location. Some therapists operate a sliding scale for older and unemployed people. Crystals themselves can cost anything from a few pence to thousands of pounds. An attractive crystal to wear as a pendant will cost about £10.

Dance movement and drama therapy

Dance movement therapy enables people to express themselves creatively through dance and movement and so help them to improve relationships, work through their difficulties and to develop strength. The psychotherapists Carl Jung and Wilhelm Reich both used expressive movement as a tool. However, dance movement therapy combines the art form of dance and movement with several psychotherapeutic models. As it is practised today it has evolved from the theories of Rudolph Laban and Mary Wigman, who were dancers and choreographers at the beginning of the twentieth century and who influenced young dancers who became pioneers of dance movement therapy in the 1940s. Drama therapy is the use of theatrical techniques and methods in a clinical or educational context, and was developed in the UK by the actress Marian 'Billy' Lindkvist. Drama and movement are sometimes used together as a therapy, or they may be used in conjunction with physiotherapy and occupational therapy.

Dance movement therapy is used to support people who are physically, mentally, emotionally or socially disadvantaged. Dance movement therapists work with adults and children of all ages and abilities with a wide range of problems such as physical disabilities, sensory difficulties, emotional/behavioural difficulties and autism, anxiety, depression, eating disorders, psychoses, bereavement, abuse, addiction and post-traumatic stress. 'Healthy' people can also find that unchoreographed movement enhances their personal communication skills, self-understanding and general feeling of wellbeing. Dance therapy is not about teaching dance technique, and participants do not require dance skills. Classes start with loosening up, and creating body awareness and emotional awareness in a way that feels natural and comfortable. The initial focus is on developing a trusting relationship; in time, movement becomes the form. Therapists may work in a circle, with rhythm, storytelling through movement, posture, gesture, movement patterns and shapes. Sometimes music is used to encourage movement; at other times the feet, hands and legs make the rhythm. Dance movement therapists work in private practice as well as in health, education and social service settings, and with individuals or groups.

Drama therapy is usually used to help people with physical disabilities, learning difficulties or eating disorders. Drama therapists work with families, groups or individuals in hospitals, day-care centres, special schools, prisons and psychiatric hospitals. Patients may be encouraged to act out a number of characters and explore different parts of their personality, which are given expression through the text. The therapist uses different theatre genres, such as melodrama, comedy or ancient Greek, to suit an individual or group.

Finding a practitioner

There are around 200 members of professional bodies in drama therapy and dance movement therapy; both these therapies are recognised by the Department of Health and have clear career structures. Indeed, both the Association for Dance Movement Therapy* and the British Association of Drama Therapists* require their practitioners to be graduates in dance or drama respectively, or in an allied subject, such as psychology. Drama therapy is available on the NHS. You will probably need to attend a session once a week for an hour. The course of treatment is individually assessed and may vary from a short course of ten weeks to a longer period depending on the person's needs. Private sessions cost between £25 and £35. Rates can vary considerably, depending on where the practitioner lives and his or her qualifications.

Feldenkrais method

The Feldenkrais method is an educational process aimed at giving people an opportunity to learn to function more easily and efficiently. It comprises a series of exercises designed to facilitate awareness of the body in movement, to improve flexibility and to enhance well-being, combined with touch and gentle manipulation. It was developed in the 1940s by Moshe Feldenkrais, who was a mechanical engineer and judo teacher. The aim with this method is to relearn healthy ways of moving and unlearn dysfunctional movement habits.

Feldenkrais practitioners believe that our posture and movement reflect the state of our nervous systems, and aim to improve physical and mental health by helping us reprogram how we move. There are two approaches used. One is known as 'functional integration', which uses individually tailored touch and manipulation on a one-to-one basis. The other is called 'awareness through movement', which is a series of simple exercises designed to help you develop body awareness and increased flexibility. These exercises are taught in groups and are popular with performers.

The Feldenkrais method is suitable for people of any age and fitness level. It is often used to treat disabilities sustained after injury, disease or a degenerative disorder and also to help with anxiety and other psychological and stress-related disorders. There are positive reports of the benefits of work by Feldenkrais himself with people with severe disabilities such as cerebral palsy; however, there are no clinical trials of the method.

Finding a practitioner

The Feldenkrais Guild UK★ has a register of trained practitioner/ teachers, who have completed a part-time training of three to four years with a minimum of 160 days' training during this time. For costs contact the individual practitioners.

Flotation therapy

Flotation therapy is a form of sensory deprivation in which your mind and body are isolated from external stimuli. The aim is to help you reach a deeply relaxed state. It was developed during the 1970s by a US neurophysiologist and psychoanalyst called Dr John Lilly, initially so that he could research how the human brain reacted when it was cut off from external simulation.

Flotation therapy involves lying in a tank filled with salty water. It is said to help relieve stress, to induce relaxation, to help people with drug problems, and to benefit people with arthritis and low back pain. Flotation tanks are found in health clubs or in specially designed float centres. The tanks are about 2.5m (8ft) long and 1.25m (4ft) wide, with about 25cm (10in) of water that contains salt to counteract gravity and is kept at skin temperature. Flotation takes place in complete or semi-darkness and with no sound; you are usually given earplugs to use. However, it is always possible to switch a light on and open the door. Sometimes, it is possible to play relaxation tapes and many tanks have a two-way microphone to enable you to talk to a practitioner, for example of hypnotherapy or psychotherapy. You can float either naked or wearing a swimming costume.

There is good scientific evidence that flotation therapy can reduce the levels of stress hormones in the body and affect our state of mind, producing a profound state of relaxation. During flotation, the brain has also been shown to release endorphins (natural opiates), which have pain-relieving properties and can produce mild feelings of euphoria. It is important to have professional supervision during flotation if you suffer from claustrophobia (and possibly other phobias), depression or anxiety. It is not suitable for people with a history of psychosis.

Finding a flotation tank

To find out where your nearest flotation tank is contact the Floatation Tank Association*. A flotation session lasts about from one to two hours. For prices contact the individual practitioners.

Flower remedies

Flower remedies, or flower essences, are specially prepared plant infusions that are used to lift the spirits, rather than to treat any under-lying symptoms. The principle behind using flower remedies is that our emotions have a strong effect on our physical condition, and lifting our mood with flower remedies should improve our health. Flower remedies were originally devised in the 1930s by Edward Bach (pronounced 'batch'), a doctor, bacteriologist and homeopath, who discovered that when he became stressed he was attracted to particular flowers, which seemed to restore his inner peace.

Flower remedies, of which the Bach Flower Remedies are the best known, are 'extracted' from the flowers of wild plants, bushes and trees by soaking sun-exposed flower heads in spring water for a few hours or by boiling the more woody plants in water. The resulting tincture, which is then preserved in brandy, is taken internally.

Dr Bach originally devised 38 remedies in total that, according to him, used in combination cover all possible states of mind. Many other flower essences are now available, such as the Bush flower essences. Some of these new essences were extracted by an American, Richard Katz, in the 1970s, since when essences from all over the world, most notably Australia, California and the Himalayas, have been developed. These are separate systems to that devised by Dr Bach, using different plants, and may have a different effect.

Bach flower remedies are said to help alleviate emotional and stress-related conditions and physical symptoms arising from emotional problems. They are not used for specific physical problems as such, but the aim is to 'balance' the emotions so that the body is free to heal itself. Bach divided his 38 remedies into seven therapeutic groups according to the following emotions: depression, fearfulness, lack of interest in the present, loneliness, over-concern with the welfare of others, over-sensitivity and uncertainty. He claimed that the remedies work through their 'energy'.

Although the Bach flower remedies are quite specific, some can be used for a variety of emotions. Chicory, for instance, is given for selfishness and possessiveness and willow is recommended for resentment and a tendency to blame others for everything, while star of Bethlehem is used for shock and feelings of loss and is a vital ingredient in Rescue Remedy. This is a mixture of five remedies with which Dr Bach allegedly saved a fisherman's life in 1930. The purpose of Rescue Remedy is to 'comfort, reassure and calm those who have received serious news, suffered a severe upset, or had a startling experience, consequently falling into a numbed, bemused state of mind'.

Dr Bach primarily developed his remedies for self-help use, and you can buy the flower remedies in many pharmacies and health food shops to treat yourself. To take Bach flower remedies, dilute two drops of remedy in a glass of water and sip the drink as and when you need it; if there is no water handy the remedy can be dropped neat on the tongue. You can take up to seven remedies at the same time. Flower remedies can also be applied directly to the skin, added to creams or lotions; put into the bath; or dispersed into the air using a spray bottle. Few complementary therapists use flower remedies alone; most practitioners who use them in their work are qualified in another therapy, such as naturopathy, aromatherapy or reflexology, or are conventionally qualified healthcare practitioners. The appropriate flower remedies can be chosen by focusing on the key emotional issues that need addressing. This was the method recommended by Dr Bach as it enables the remedies to be understood and used by everyone. Some people, however, prefer to select remedies by using intuition, kinesiology or dowsing.

Scientific analyses of flower remedies show that there is nothing in them apart from alcohol and spring water – though numerous anecdotes report success with flower remedies. Very few clinical trials exist to show that they work, and the trials that have been conducted have been of poor quality or yielded conflicting results. In fact, the only two rigorous trials were negative. Despite this paucity of evidence, a surprising number of people, including medical practitioners, swear by flower remedies. This could be due to the placebo effect, or the brandy in which the tincture is preserved, although the latter is very unlikely as only a few drops, diluted in water, are taken. Flower remedies are harmless and can be taken by anyone of any age or condition, even animals.

Finding a practitioner

One of the attractions of flower remedies is that a lay person can easily treat him- or herself with them, unlike, say, herbs and homeopathic remedies, which ideally require trained practitioners to dispense them. If you want to visit a practitioner, contact the Dr Edward Bach Centre*, which keeps a list of around 1,000 therapists who have successfully completed its three-stage course and have signed the Bach Foundation's code of ethics and practice. The Centre will also give free advice over the phone. Flower remedies are fairly cheap: a 10ml bottle costs around £3; a 20ml bottle £6. Advice from a practitioner registered with the Bach Foundation will cost about £25.

Hellerwork

This therapy combines deep tissue bodywork, movement education and exploration of emotional issues. It is primarily used for conditions which may be caused or exacerbated by a person's posture. This could include chronic back pain, headaches or stress-related problems. Many people embrace Hellerwork as a way of reconnecting with their bodies, in a world which is very brain-orientated. An American engineer, Joseph Heller, developed the therapy in the 1970s after training as a rolfer. However, he decided that simply restructuring the body with deep tissue massage, as is the case with rolfing, would not produce lasting effects. He took the rolfing ideas about body alignment and releasing muscular tension a stage further by integrating movement awareness and dialogue about psychoemotional issues with the bodywork.

The thinking behind Hellerwork is that the body is a hologram of the whole being, manifesting our physical and emotional habit patterns as well as any trauma in its structure. This needs to be brought to awareness and released to get lasting benefit from deep tissue massage. A course of Hellerwork comprises 11 sessions, each lasting around 90 minutes. During this time, the practitioner will use deep pressure and manipulation to realign the soft tissue of the body, as well as 'movement re-education' or special exercises that help to bring increased awareness to your body usage and teach you stress-free ways to perform everyday activities. The practitioner will also use dialogue to encourage the expression of any emotions or memories that are triggered by the release of body tensions.

Deep tissue bodywork is designed to release any tension in your connective tissue, and to realign the body. The practitioner works with his or her hands to release tension in the fascia, to create more suppleness and flexibility in the tissue and more space and fluidity in the movement of the joints. Bodywork accounts for about 60 minutes of each session. Movement education aims to enable you to become profoundly aware of your body and your movement patterns in daily activities and, as a result, to discover easier, fuller ways of moving. Simple and easy to remember suggestions and visualisations are used to help you rebalance your movement and gain optimal alignment and fluidity. The practitioner will work with you while you are sitting, standing, walking and performing other common movements and movements particular to you, such as those of your favourite sport, or your job activity. Video feedback is sometimes used to assist the movement education process, and to allow you to get a picture of how your body moves from the outside. The verbal dialogue component of Hellerwork focuses on allowing you to become aware of the relationship between your emotions and attitudes and your body, so that they are less likely to limit your body and your self-expression.

In each session, a different part of the body is focused on. For example, session one focuses on the chest and the theme in the verbal dialogue component is 'Inspiration'. The 11 sessions are divided into three groups to facilitate a layer-by-layer release of tension and held-in trauma from the body. The first group comprises the superficial sessions, which focus on the surface of the body's connective tissue and those muscles near the surface of the body. Developmentally, these superficial sessions deal with issues of infancy and childhood, such as breathing, standing up, and reaching out. The second group comprises the core sessions, which concentrate on the deeper muscles and connective tissue of the body. The core muscles help us in fine motor movements and so help us to move with grace and fluidity. These sessions focus on development issues of adolescence such as control and surrender, gut feelings, holding back feelings and intellectual development. The integrative sessions are designed to integrate the superficial and the core sessions, and the practitioner aims to balance and align the unique patterns of each client's body. The final, eleventh, session does not necessarily include bodywork and seeks to combine the Hellerwork series with your entire life. Developmentally, the integrative sessions focus on issues of maturity such as masculine and feminine styles and values, integration and coming out into the world.

Hellerworkers claim that when you complete a Hellerwork series your body is in a new state of alignment, is much more balanced and much freer in movement. People report that their bodies continue to change for some time as a result of the Hellerwork series, perhaps for as long as a year. Hellerworkers recommend that you have a follow-up session after any kind of trauma, physical or emotional, during which the practitioner can focus on rebalancing your entire body. There has been little scientific research carried out on Hellerwork. One uncontrolled study of employees in a computer software company found that it improved posture and reduced physical stress and back pain. Most of the employees also reported that it helped improve their working relationships. However, the study was poorly designed. Do not have Hellerwork therapy if you have cancer, rheumatoid arthritis or any other inflammatory conditions.

Finding a practitioner

There are very few qualified Hellerworkers in the UK. To find a certified practitioner, contact Hellerwork International★ or the European Hellerwork Association★. Certified Hellerwork practitioners

(CHP) complete 1,250 hours of study and once certified must follow a code of ethics, sexual conduct policy, communicable disease policy and a procedure for mediation and resolution. They must also participate in approved continuing professional education and maintain liability insurance. For prices of a course of Hellerwork contact the individual practitioners.

Holotropic breathwork

Holotropic breathwork uses a combination of breathing and music to induce an altered state of consciousness, in which emotional and physical healing, and personal and spiritual growth, are reputed to take place. It was developed by the psychiatrist Stanislav Grof in the USA in the 1960s. Evidence from cave paintings suggests that altered states of consciousness have been used by human beings for up to 40,000 years in rituals and spiritual practices. Dr Grof developed holotropic breathwork from a wide range of ancient methods for accessing these states of consciousness, such as Buddhist and Hindu breathing techniques and traditional music from indigenous peoples the world over.

Originally, Dr Grof conducted research into the use of the hallucinogenic drug LSD in psychotherapy. During this research, he found that when the participants were in an altered state of consciousness due to the drug, the reality of their inner world was very different from external reality. In this altered state, they reported re-experiencing past events such as physical or emotional traumas, that issues of death and rebirth emerged strongly and that they seemed to relive their own births. Some of their experiences even seemed spiritual or paranormal, such as having contact with mythological figures, deities and spirit guides, experiencing past lives, or having access to knowledge from other cultures or times, and a sense of connection with other people, species or the whole universe. These experiences are called transpersonal because they transcend the usual boundaries of personality. Dr Grof's work with LSD was very controversial, however, and he went on to see if there was some other way to create similar states of consciousness and these transpersonal experiences. What emerged was a technique that involves rapid breathing, supported by the use of carefully chosen music, to access altered states of consciousness.

A holotropic breathwork session usually takes place in a group and lasts two to three hours. Before you start 'breathing', you should be given an introductory talk that explains how you can get the most out of the session. People work in pairs, taking it in turns to be the 'breather' and the 'helper'. The helper is expected to give undivided and non-judgemental attention to the 'breather' and attend to their needs. When you are breathing, you start off lying on your back with your eyes closed and are talked through progressive muscle relaxation to help you relax. Then you will be instructed to increase your rate and depth of breathing as the music starts, while keeping your awareness on your inner experiences. The aim of the music is to help you move through any blocks that come up during the session. The rapid breathing, in effect, creates hyperventilation, which holotropic breathworkers claim allows deep-seated tensions and patterns to surface. You may shake, twitch, cough, vomit, sweat or verbalise your experience with words or sounds, and this is interpreted as spontaneous release of these patterns. Some people also experience prolonged muscular contractions and spasms; others experience heightened sensory awareness, ecstatic states or sexual feelings. Some people move around a lot or even dance, while others stay absolutely still. If you experience symptoms such as pain, numbness, cold or heat in the body, your helper or the breathworker running the group, with your consent, can use some form of pressure to help amplify the sensation. After the breathing, you will be encouraged to do some art, such as a drawing or painting, to represent your experience. The aim is to help you integrate your experience. There will usually be an opportunity for group sharing after everyone has completed their 'breathe'. If you find the prospect of a group session daunting, it is possible to arrange individual sessions.

Anecdotally, people claim that holotropic breathwork has resulted in dramatic changes in long-standing medical problems such as chronic pain, asthma or eczema, in relief of mental and emotional problems such as anxiety or phobias, and in deeper spiritual awareness and enhanced creativity. No formal scientific research has been carried out on the effectiveness of holotropic breathwork. It is safe for most people, but is not suitable for people with heart or circulatory conditions or glaucoma, if you have had recent surgery or an injury, or if you are pregnant. If you have epilepsy, check with your doctor first and, while holotropic breathwork can be beneficial for people with a history of mental illness, it is only appropriate in the context of residential or intensive outpatient support from appropriately trained healthcare practitioners.

Rebirthing, which was developed by Leonard Orr in the 1960s, has some similarities to holotropic breathwork, except that it uses what is called 'conscious connected breathing'. This involves learning to breathe in a circular way with no pause between the inhalation and the exhalation and no holding of air in the lungs. Rebirthing uses this type of breathing to move you into non-ordinary states of consciousness. It is used to bring suppressed experiences from the past, and memories of birth and even past lives to the surface. During a rebirth the rebirther works in a psychotherapeutic way with you to help you accept and integrate your experiences into your present life.

Finding a practitioner

There is currently only a handful of certified holotropic breathworkers in the UK. The training currently involves 500 hours of experiential work, lectures and apprenticeship over a minimum of two years. Members of the Association of Holotropic Breathwork International all subscribe to an agreed code of ethics. To find out more about rebirthing contact the British Rebirth Society*, which has a code of ethics and practice, and works to maintain the standards of rebirthing in the UK.

Light therapy

Light therapy is used both in complementary and conventional medicine. In conventional medicine, where it is known as phototherapy, it is used to treat jaundice in newborns and, as PUVA (UV light combined with a drug called psoralens), to treat psoriasis. In complementary medicine, light therapy is used to treat seasonal affective disorder (SAD), which is a type of depression that some people get in the winter and is thought to be caused by light deprivation, and also to treat insomnia and disturbed sleep patterns (for example, due to night shifts or jet lag).

The benefits of natural sunlight have probably been known for centuries. In the nineteenth century, patients in sanatoriums were advised to exercise regularly in bright sunlight, and incandescent electric light baths were used to treat a range of physical and mental illnesses. More recently, scientists have realised the important role that light plays in regulating the body's biological clock or biorhythms. It is now known that the body has what is called circadian rhythms that match the 24-hour solar day. For example, blood pressure, body temperature, the urinary excretion of potassium and cortisol secretion are all at their highest during the day, while levels of melatonin (a hormone that is involved in our sleeping patterns) and white blood cells are at their highest at night. The study of these biorhythms is called chronobiology. Light plays its part in our body rhythms by stimulating nerve impulses to the brain when it enters the eyes. These nerve impulses travel to the hypothalamus, the part of the brain responsible for appetite, sleep, mood, temperature and sex drive, and the pineal gland in the brain, which regulates hormones such as serotonin, a hormone linked to mood, and melatonin.

Artificial bright light therapy was developed at the US National Institute of Mental Health in the early 1980s and was first used to treat people with SAD. Research found that they needed to be exposed to the high intensity light for two to six hours daily to gain any benefit. Although the improvement seen was dramatic, it was not feasible for working people to spend this amount of time under a lamp. New lamps were developed that were effective if used for about 30 to 45 minutes daily. These are positioned about 30cm (12in) away from the eyes on a tilted stand, so that the light falls downwards towards the eyes. They emit fluorescent full-spectrum light (bright white light) that is the same as natural daylight but with the toxic UV wavelengths taken out. As such, light therapy differs from phototherapy used in conventional medicine, which retains the UV wavelengths.

Treatment with light therapy can be carried out at home using a light box. The amount of time needed to sit in front of the light and the time of day will vary from person to person, but 30 minutes of exposure daily at about 7 o'clock in the morning with 10,000 lux illumination is a good starting point for people with SAD or those who are drowsy in the mornings. Some people find this amount causes irritability or early morning awakening, and need to shorten the sessions, sit further from the light or do the treatment later in the day. Other patients will need more exposure by sitting for longer sessions (but rarely more than an hour) or do the treatment earlier. It is also possible to consult a practitioner and have the treatment in his or her practice.

Here, you would be required to lie with your eyes open on a couch under a lamp the length of your body for about an hour. These lamps emit bright white light of at least 2,500 lux.

There have been several studies to show that SAD exists and can be treated by light therapy, while there is good evidence to support the use of PUVA for psoriasis. Several mild adverse effects have been reported with light therapy, such as eye irritation and headaches, but these tend to go quickly or can be controlled by reducing exposure to light. People with progressive diseases of the retina, such as macular degeneration, should avoid light therapy and people who are taking medicines associated with photosensitisation such as tricyclic antidepressants and lithium should have their eyes checked regularly. Risks with phototherapy include direct eye injury and photosensitivity, while strobe lights can provoke seizures in susceptible individuals. It is vital to consult a properly qualified medical practitioner for PUVA treatment, because there have been recent reports of people sustaining very severe burns when they have been given a herbal product containing psoralea in conjunction with UV light therapy by a complementary therapist.

Finding a practitioner

To find a practitioner who offers light therapy, or to obtain your own light box, contact the SAD Association*.

Magnetic therapy

Magnetic therapy, also known as biomagnet therapy or magnetic field therapy, uses permanent or pulsed magnetic fields applied to the head or other parts of the body to treat disease. Strong, electro-magnetic fields are used in conventional medicine to help heal wounds and fractures. In complementary medicine, permanent weak magnetic fields are used to treat a wide range of conditions. The use of magnets in this way can be traced back to ancient civili-sations – Cleopatra is alleged to have worn a magnet on her head in an attempt to stop her ageing. It is, though, to the work of the Austrian doctor Franz Anton Mesmer, in the eighteenth century, that magnetic therapy as we know it owes its origins. He claimed that magnets could enhance what he termed 'animal magnetism', a universal force that flows through our bodies.

One theory behind magnetic therapy is that the iron atoms in red blood cells respond to magnets, so that when a magnet is placed on a person's body, blood flow through the area is increased. This, in turn, improves the supply of oxygen and nutrients to cells in the area and enhances the elimination of waste products.

Conventional medicine now recognises that strong electromagnetic fields, generated by electrical devices, can be effective in helping broken bones to heal: the Food and Drug Authority in the USA has approved its use for fractures that have failed to heal. Doctors worldwide now also use strong electromagnetic fields to treat deep vein thrombosis, oedema, osteoporosis and non-healing wounds such as leg ulcers. Magnetic resonance imaging (MRI) scans are widely used in conventional medicine to diagnose disease and are considered to be safer and more sensitive than X-rays.

Weak magnets are mainly used as a self-help therapy, for a wide variety of indications such as arthritis, back pain, headaches and migraines, insomnia and fatigue. It is possible to buy magnetic straps to wear over joints affected by arthritis; magnetic mattresses, pillows and car seat covers; magnetic shoe insoles; and even tiny 'supermagnets' on plasters. A remedy for poor digestion is magnetised water, which is made by placing a jug of water on a magnet's negative pole for about 24 hours. There is some scientific research on the effectiveness of weak magnetic fields to treat disease. The results are neither uniform nor compelling, not least because of the range of indications and the large variety of magnetic fields used (e.g. static *vs* pulsed).

Magnetic therapy should be avoided by people with pacemakers. Women who are pregnant, and people with myasthenia gravis or bleeding disorders should not go in for self-help therapy.

Finding a practitioner

Strong electromagnetic fields for fracture healing are used in a few NHS hospitals in the UK. A variety of complementary practitioners might advise that you use static magnets as part of your treatment; for example, some acupuncturists place tiny magnets on plasters over acupuncture points to supplement their treatments. Either your practitioner will show you how to use a magnet, or it will come with manufacturer's instructions. To find out more about this type of treatment or find a local practitioner, contact the British

Biomagnetic Association*, which is an organisation of practitioners (mainly acupuncturists and osteopaths).

Metamorphic technique

This technique involves gently touching specific parts of the hands, feet and head with the aim of creating an environment free of direction in which emotional and physical patterns can be released. It is founded on the belief that these patterns are established during the time spent in the womb, when our strengths and weaknesses are first determined. Releasing them is believed to lead to profound creative changes. The metamorphic technique was developed in the 1960s by a British naturopath and reflexologist, Robert St John, who worked in an institution for children with autism and Down's syndrome. He found that his work as a reflexologist was helpful, but only in the short term. The children returned to the same old patterns of ill health after treatment. He formulated the view that the only approach that would work permanently would involve the freeing of a person's own life force to do the healing.

Practitioners of the metamorphic technique claim that, by lightly touching areas along an imaginary line (called a 'time line') that runs from the ankle along the arch to the big toe, as well as parts of the hands and head, they provide a context in which the person's 'life force' can act freely. This, in turn, can alter difficult patterns laid down in the past. Practitioners feel strongly that they are not the ones doing the healing, but that they merely act as catalysts to help their patients change. They are trained to make no comment nor offer any counselling or advice. The idea is that, through the metamorphic technique, patients gain inner strength and self-esteem because they are the ones who are doing the healing and transforming their own lives.

Practitioners do not claim that the technique itself is good for any specific health problem, but that it is a person's life force that can bring about the healing. Nevertheless, people have the metamorphic technique for a variety of conditions, and it is considered particularly beneficial for people with long-term physical and mental illnesses. The metamorphic technique is also considered to be good for people with addictions because it encourages a person's 'vital energy' to fight the drugs or alcohol, thus restoring lost self-esteem.

At a session of the metamorphic technique, the practitioner gently touches the inside of the feet, hands and head, in that order, spending about half an hour on the feet, which are considered more important than the hands or head. He or she will use light stroking movements, sometimes circular, working perhaps just a few centimetres above the skin. The practitioner does not ask about your personal life or illnesses, or give advice on diet, lifestyle or anything else, as this is regarded as imposing his or her understanding on you, which is not part of the technique's philosophy.

After a session with a metamorphic technique practitioner you should feel very relaxed. A day or so later you may experience a surge of energy or feel a bit confused. Practitioners are very open about the technique, and patients are taught how to use it at home and on their families, encouraging self-help. No scientific evidence exists to prove that metamorphic technique works; indeed, gathering evidence would be against the whole approach of the technique. Because practitioners believe that people heal themselves, nothing is 'done' and therefore nothing can be tested. Nevertheless, GPs and hospital doctors are showing interest in the technique and a few have practitioners attached to their surgeries and clinics. Some GPs maintain that metamorphic technique is good for relieving stress and stress-related conditions.

Because the technique is non-invasive, it can do no harm. However, if you have a serious medical condition you should consult your GP first.

Finding a practitioner

Over 2,000 people have undergone weekend training courses given by Gaston Saint-Pierre and other teachers. He was taught the technique by St John, and he went on to establish the Metamorphic Association* in 1979, a charitable trust since 1982 which has 250 members. The aim of the association is to show people the technique so that they can return home and start using it with family and friends. It is believed that through practice they will discover the importance of detachment – as a 'catalyst', the practitioner needs to be completely detached, and this state cannot be taught, asserts Saint-Pierre, but has to be experienced. A session of metamorphic technique usually lasts an hour and costs about £30 to £55, depending on location.

Music therapy

Music therapy consists of making music for therapeutic purposes. The ancient Greeks and Egyptians used music therapy extensively, but it was during the Second World War, when music therapy was used to help soldiers traumatised by the fighting, that musicians started being employed in hospitals. Today, in the UK, music therapy is well established, with about 500 qualified music therapists, all of whom are required to be state registered with the Health Professions Council and some of whom are employed in the NHS. The therapy is used to treat psychological problems, pain, neurological disability and communication disorders.

The ability to appreciate music, which remains unimpaired by illness or injury, may be the only thing that can alleviate the pain brought on by physical or mental suffering. While music therapists are holistic in their approach to clients, they are also clinically directed and have specific aims and objectives.

Music therapists work in hospitals, special schools, day centres and prisons; are employed by the NHS, the local education authority or social services department; and may also have private practices. A music therapist often works as part of a team, alongside other practitioners, such as speech therapists, occupational therapists or physiotherapists, as well as doctors.

Music therapy is mostly active, in which a patient or group of patients plays musical instruments and/or sings, and the therapist takes an active part in such sessions by listening and responding by playing or singing. The aim of active music therapy is to help express emotions in non-verbal ways and to release tension, so that you are able to deal more effectively with any problems you have. During a session, you are not taught how to play an instrument; rather, you are encouraged to use percussion and other musical instruments to create a musical language and the therapist will usually improvise together with you. An active music session usually lasts about an hour. Music therapy can sometimes involve playing music for people to listen to. It can, for example, reduce anxiety in people waiting for surgery or help people on intensive care, coronary care and cancer units to relax. Its aim is to gradually improve mood, reducing anxiety and lifting depression.

For people who find verbal communication difficult and who may be isolated and withdrawn, music therapy can be enormously beneficial. For someone whose difficulties are largely emotional, creating music can be a safe way to express and release all kinds of emotions. Research shows that music therapy is particularly beneficial for children and adults with physical and learning disabilities. Many studies have shown that music relaxes people and improves their mood. Recent studies have also shown that it can relieve the anxiety and fear that exacerbate pain.

Finding a practitioner

The Association of Professional Music Therapists★ and the British Society for Music Therapy★ both have details of qualified music therapists, who can be recognised by the letters RMTh (Registered Music Therapist) or SRMTh (State Registered Music Therapist) after their names. Music therapists have to be trained musicians and are required to undergo one of the UK's recognised training courses. For prices contact individual practitioners.

Polarity therapy

Dr Randolph Stone, a naturopath, osteopath and chiropractor, developed polarity therapy in the mid-twentieth century. Dr Stone also studied Eastern systems of healing and drew on elements from Traditional Chinese Medicine, Ayurveda, his own practice and conventional medicine in an attempt to create an all-encompassing healing system, which he named polarity therapy. Essentially, it is an energy-based system and polarity therapists use their hands to influence the flow of 'energy' around the body. They also give verbal support throughout the treatment and advise on special stretching exercises and nutrition. Polarity therapy is used to treat anxiety, stress, other psychological problems, migraines, chronic fatigue syndrome, pre-menstrual syndrome, allergies, irritable bowel syndrome, back pain and arthritis.

Polarity therapists claim to work with the 'human energy field', the electromagnetic patterns expressed in mental, emotional and physical experience. Health is viewed as a reflection of the condition of this energy field, and the therapy is designed to balance the field to improve health and well-being. Dr Stone found that the 'human energy field' is affected by touch, diet, movement, sound, attitudes, relationships, life experience, trauma and environmental factors. Good health is experienced when the energy flows smoothly around the body. When it is unbalanced, depleted, blocked or fixed due to stress or other factors, pain and disease are said to arise. Therapists believe that energy is kept in constant motion by the pull of opposing poles in the body, which act like magnets. The left side of the body and feet are the negative pole and the right side and head are the positive pole, with the centre of the body being neutral.

Underlying principles of polarity therapy are that: the practitioner's hands are conductors of energy; people respond to the consciousness of the practitioner as well as his or her touch; by creating an environment of safety and recognition, the practitioner supports the patient's self-healing process; energy can be palpated by both practitioner and patient; and everyone has a subconscious inner intelligence and self-regulating capacity, which emerges with awareness of energy movement.

In a typical polarity therapy session, the practitioner first assesses your energy by asking you about your health, medical history, family history, lifestyle and diet. You will then be asked to lie on a couch while the practitioner assesses your energy using touch, and 'balances' your energy by applying concentrated pressure on specific points on the body with the aim of realigning posture and improving the flow of energy around the body. The pressure may be light, medium or firm. You will not need to undress for the treatment. During the session, the practitioner may use verbal skills to support the client's increasing self-awareness of subtle energetic sensations, which are often experienced as tingling, warmth, expansion or wavelike movement. The verbal support might include describing specific links between the body and emotions using models such as the chakras and Yin and Yang to do so, and also might support patients in taking charge of their lives, finding their own solutions and managing stress. The therapist may also suggest some polarity yoga exercises for you to do for a few minutes every day at home. The postures are reminiscent of the techniques of traditional hatha yoga and related systems, but are generally easier to do and are specifically designed to balance energy and are accompanied by gentle rocking and vocal expressions. The aim of the yoga is to strengthen the spine, tone and stretch muscles, improve the flow of energy and release toxins. Finally, polarity therapy puts a strong emphasis on the importance of nutrition and advocates a diet containing lots of fresh fruit and vegetables. Advice is based on the energetic properties of foods, in contrast to nutritional systems that measure specific components such as vitamin and mineral content. In addition, polarity therapy uses foods for specific beneficial effects, particularly cleansing and rebuilding the body using high-energy foods, herbal foods, food combining (that is, never eating proteins at the same time as carbohydrates) and detoxifying diets. A great emphasis is put on self-help and personal responsibility, and you will be encouraged to take charge of your health. If the practitioner thinks that you have negative thoughts that are contributing to your health problems, you may be advised to have counselling to encourage a positive attitude and to enhance your self-esteem.

Anecdotally, the results of polarity therapy vary, and may include profound relaxation, new insight into energetic patterns and their implications, release of held-in emotions and relief from numerous specific problems. No clinical trials have been conducted to assess the effectiveness of polarity therapy. There are no known safety concerns with polarity therapy, although elimination and detoxifying diets should only be undertaken with professional supervision.

Finding a practitioner

Polarity therapy is mainly practised in the USA and the American Polarity Therapy Association (APTA), which was set up in 1984, has over 150 registered practitioners. The APTA publishes the Polarity Therapy Standards for Practice and its Code of Ethics, and has set the foundation for the training certification of practitioners and schools. The UK Polarity Therapy Association★ and the Federation of Polarity Training★ maintain a register of practitioners in the UK and offer training through the International School of Polarity Therapy, which comprises 20 weekend workshops over a two-year period or an intensive one-year training, one day a week. Contact an individual practitioner to find out how much a session costs; each session will take 60–90 minutes.

Rolfing

Rolfing, which is also known as structural integration, was developed by Dr Ida Rolf, an American biochemist. It involves pressure and manipulation of connective tissue as well as education in movement. The aim is to release stress patterns, and enable you to move and function with greater freedom, and effortlessly maintain a more upright posture.

Dr Rolf spent over 50 years studying the bodily structure of thousands of people, and came to the conclusion that chronic poor posture was caused by shortened connective tissue around the muscles and that physical efficiency was at its peak when the major segments of the body (the head, shoulders, abdomen, pelvis and legs) were aligned and balanced in a specific way. She then discovered that skilful manipulation could lengthen the shortened connective tissue, and developed a system that became known as the Rolf Method of Structural Integration. In the early 1960s, in response to demand, she began to teach her technique. Today, there are about 700 practitioners who carry on her work throughout the world.

Rolfing practitioners believe that our bodies are in constant battle with the pull of gravity, and that this is made worse by the stresses and strains of life. They also believe that poor posture affects our emotional and physical well-being, and results in more energy expenditure to keep the body in an upright position. According to rolfing practitioners, the connective tissue throughout our bodies unites a set of relationships that are characteristic of a particular individual. Their aim is to work with the human structure via connective tissue, in such a way that the different parts of the body move and fit together in an improved relationship to each other and within the Earth's gravitational field. Rolfing is designed to lengthen and release connective tissue, which in turn is said to improve blood flow and eliminate energy loss caused by muscle strain. Once you have been 'rolfed' it might look as though you are simply standing a bit straighter. However, rolfers say their technique does not just improve posture, but that it allows the body to re-align itself with gravity, helping the individual to function better and allowing the body's natural healing powers to work unimpeded.

A basic course of rolfing consists of ten sessions, each lasting about one hour. At the first session, the practitioner will take your case history, and may take a photograph or video of you from the front, back and sides for analysis later. You may be asked to stand in front of a mirror and try to look at your body through the eyes of the practitioner. As with osteopathy and chiropractic, you will be asked to undress down to your underwear. Then, while you lie on a massage couch, the practitioner will apply pressure with his or her fingers, hands, knuckles or elbows to smooth out your connective tissue.

Each session focuses on a different part of the body. In the first session, for instance, the practitioner might concentrate on the shoulders, chest, lower back and pelvis; in the second on the area from the knees to the feet, and so on. Rolfing is not a particularly relaxing experience. It is sometimes uncomfortable, and even painful. Practitioners claim that the pain is due to the connective tissue releasing and that it should only last for a few seconds. However, you may feel a bit sore for a few days after a rolfing session. People who have experienced severe emotional trauma or women who are pregnant should approach rolfing with caution. It is not appropriate for people who bruise very easily, those with osteoporosis, cancer or rheumatoid arthritis, or for people who are obese.

Anecdotally, rolfing is said to result in a feeling of improved fitness, vigour and well-being. People who have had a course of rolfing claim that they can stand taller, with more stability and less strain, breathe deeper and more easily, and move with more naturalness and grace. Many also say that they feel more supple after a rolfing session. Some people have reported that they can sense an emotional release after treatment.

Rolfing practitioners do not claim that it can cure disease, but do say that it can help with neck pain, back problems, impaired mobility and other difficulties that can arise from chronic stress and tension, such as irritable bowel syndrome, period pains and anxiety. Some people have it to improve their appearance, increase their athletic or artistic performance, or to further personal growth towards a fuller realisation of their potential. One small randomised controlled trial found that rolfing was better than no intervention for reducing anxiety, while another found that it helped to correct curvature of the spine.

Finding a practitioner

There are only a handful of qualified rolfing practitioners in the UK. Training can be completed in one year, in four intensive units. For details of qualified UK practitioners, contact the Rolf Institute★. It should cost you about £50 for each session.

Sound therapy

Sound therapy, or sound healing, is different from music therapy – it involves the rhythmic use of sound to 'recharge' the brain with energy in a similar way to Buddhist chanting or the Muslim call to prayer. Doctors first become interested in the healing potential of sound in the late nineteenth century, when researchers in the USA found that different types of music could increase mental clarity and stimulate blood flow, but it was in the mid-twentieth century that machines were developed that used sound waves as a form of therapy.

Today, sound is used on many different levels. In conventional medicine, ultrasound waves are used to break up kidney stones, to stimulate healing or as a diagnostic technique. Sound therapy is used by healthy people to 'widen their consciousness', and as a complementary therapy to treat learning difficulties, dyslexia and autism, mental and emotional problems such as depression and anxiety, high blood pressure and musculoskeletal pain.

There are several different ways in which you can experience sound therapy. Some practitioners use the voice, such as through chanting, others use electronic or musical instruments to generate sound waves. You can attend a day or weekend workshop, and learn how to chant from a repertoire of native American, Tibetan or Mongolian chants. Sometimes, the therapist will also use drums in these workshops. Sound healers claim that chanting makes you still, centred, alert, empowered and relaxed.

Another method that is growing in popularity in the UK is the Tomatis method, which uses a machine to transmit certain sound frequencies. This was developed by Dr Alfred Tomatis, a Paris-based ear, nose and throat specialist, who was one of the first people to investigate the auditory environment of the foetus. His theory was that the auditory relationship between baby and mother lays the foundation for all our other relationships and is therefore the crucial point of intervention to bring about change in the person's psychological response to sound and language. In the 1940s, Dr Tomatis devised a system of taking the listener back through the auditory experience of being in the womb and first learning to identify sound. He called this process 'sonic birth'. He initially concerned himself with hearing loss. When someone has hearing loss it is usually partial, not total, and in a particular frequency. Dr Tomatis designed an apparatus called the 'Electronic Ear', which could boost the deficient frequencies in a person with hearing loss to enable him or her to hear normally again.

The Tomatis approach involves listening to specially recorded analogue tapes of highly filtered classical music. This is said to stimulate the ear and the brain by presenting it with constantly alternating sounds of high and low tone. With this approach, the sound must be listened to on a cassette player that reaches a frequency response of at least 16,000 Hertz (16 Kilohertz), and through headphones (or earphones), not through speakers. A portable player is highly recommended as it allows you to move around and so manage the required hours of listening without interfering with your daily activities. Ideally, the player should be auto-reverse, so that you can listen while asleep. The required listening time is three hours a day for adults and 30 to 60 minutes a day for children. It can take anything from a few days to a few months to see some results, but on average the programme takes between six weeks and three months to achieve full results. However, sound therapy is played at very low volume on portable equipment so you can listen while performing your usual daily activities; while listening, you can read, work, exercise, talk, listen to the radio, watch TV, have a conversation, talk on the phone, use a computer or even sleep.

Auditory integration training, which was developed by Dr Guy Berard, is similar to the Tomatis approach, while physio-acoustic methodology, which was designed in Finland, uses computer-generated sound waves played through speakers in a special chair.

Health claims for the Tomatis approach include: improved vitality and well-being; deep relaxation and relief of anxiety; heightened creativity, improved concentration and learning ability; increased energy, focus and performance; relief of insomnia; improved hearing for those with industrial deafness or hearing loss due to ageing; relief of tinnitus; improved balance and recovery from Menière's vertigo; recovery from learning problems such as

attention deficit hyperactivity disorder and dyslexia; and better relationships, improved communication and greater family harmony.
Very few studies of sound therapy have been conducted, though two
small pilot studies, one of the Tomatis approach, the other of
auditory integration training, found that they may be beneficial in
people with behavioural problems.

Finding a practitioner

There are a number of training schools throughout the world,
which offer varying degrees of training. Often, sound therapists
have a musical background and some are trained in another complementary therapy. A day's sound therapy workshop will cost
anything from £25–£100 and a weekend can cost anything from
£80 upwards. Contact the Listening Centre UK Ltd★ for more
information about the Tomatis approach.

T'ai chi and qigong

Westerners visiting China in the early 1970s were fascinated to see
parks full of people at the crack of dawn exercising as if in a slow-
motion film: now, nearly every adult education institute in the UK
has a t'ai chi class. Qigong is less well known here but is growing in
popularity. Part of Traditional Chinese Medicine, it is an ancient
system of meditational movements and actually forms the basis for
t'ai chi and other Eastern therapeutic exercise systems. T'ai chi is
sometimes described as a dynamic form of qigong. Both qigong and
t'ai chi involve simple movements that are designed to boost and
balance Qi (energy) in our bodies.

T'ai chi is a martial art: it is actually a type of kung fu. However,
it is 'non-violent' and has no competitive edge. T'ai chi, or *t'ai chi
chuan* (*t'ai chi* means 'the supreme unity' and *chuan* the 'fist' or
'container'), to give it its full name, comprises a series of postures
linked by gentle, graceful movements. The set series are called
forms, and are designed to bring about good health and well-being
by restoring the natural flow of Qi within the body. The movements
are said to be a way of stabilising the two opposing and fluctuating
forces of Yin and Yang, which are believed to reflect the ebb and
flow of life. The exercises were inspired by the natural movements
of nature – the wind, birds in flight, the sea, etc.

T'ai chi is usually taught in groups, for two reasons. First, you need someone to demonstrate the movements, and second, it can take some time to learn them (between six months and three years to gain any proficiency and very much longer to master the movements completely). However, with a good teacher, subtle benefits can be experienced after a few lessons. There are a number of different styles and forms of t'ai chi. Today, the two most commonly taught forms are known as the 'short form' and the 'long form'. The short form consists of 24 movements that can be performed in about ten minutes; the 'long form' takes 20–40 minutes and comprises 108 movements. The movements are slow, pleasurable and linked, so that one flows into another.

Qigong is a branch of Traditional Chinese Medicine that uses posture, breathing and meditation to increase awareness and control of Qi. Literally translated, qigong means 'energy cultivation'. As well as being used in a similar way to t'ai chi to help maintain good health, well-being and energy, it is also used therapeutically. Qigong movements, of which there are thousands, can be learnt in a class or you can visit a qigong master for treatment and to learn the movements. The teacher will help you learn to recognise sensations of Qi and to use your mind to guide it in certain beneficial ways. Unlike in t'ai chi, the exercises in qigong can be practised in any order. Qigong masters are said to be able to transmit Qi into other people in order to heal them. Qigong is used to treat a wide range of health problems.

People who practice t'ai chi report that the concentration and discipline needed to remember the forms still the mind, and the steady breathing has a calming effect. Some doctors recommend t'ai chi to patients who have heart problems and high blood pressure. Clinical trials have shown that t'ai chi appears to improve balance and strength in older people, and to reduce the risk of falls. Trials have also shown that it may help with depression and tiredness and may improve the function of the heart and lungs in older people. There has been little formal research of qigong. However, one observational study that followed up more than 1,000 people with high blood pressure for at least 20 years found that, during the study, 17 per cent of the people who had practised qigong died compared to 32 per cent of those who had not practised qigong. Case studies report that qigong can help people with asthma, arthritis, digestive tract problems, insomnia, pain, depression, anxiety, heart disease or cancer.

Both t'ai chi and qigong are suitable for people of any age, for those with disabilities such as multiple sclerosis and polio, and for those recovering from illness or injuries. Although they are usually performed standing, they can be adapted for wheelchair-users, who reputedly gain much benefit. Qigong has been reported to trigger psychosis, probably in those who have it as an underlying condition. It is possible to sustain injuries such as a sprain or a strain while practising t'ai chi or qigong.

Finding a teacher

T'ai chi teachers should have a basic understanding of human anatomy and physiology, and have certified knowledge of first aid in medical emergencies. Ideally, they will have studied with a master before teaching, and have had at least five years of personal experience of t'ai chi. Many local authorities, local adult evening classes and health clubs offer t'ai chi lessons; a class will cost you about £5 to £10. Some t'ai chi schools run drop-in classes, but you need to have a course of at least ten sessions to get any benefit. Finding a qigong teacher or master is less easy, as there are still relatively few in the UK. For more information, contact The Qigong Centre*: qigong teachers/masters usually train with a master for many years.

Tragerwork

The Trager approach was developed by Dr Milton Trager in the USA over a period of 65 years. As a teenager Dr Trager was interested in boxing, body-building, acrobatics and dancing. He trained as a physiotherapist and then as a doctor and went on to combine his experiences to create Tragerwork. This involves gentle movements performed by the therapist plus training in self-help movement therapy. Dr Trager set up the Trager Institute in 1980.

The aim of Tragerwork is to reintegrate the body and mind and to release deep-seated patterns, so helping improve health and well-being. It is used in many chronic physical and psychological conditions, particularly those that are associated with or aggravated by stress. There are two aspects to Tragerwork; one in which you are passive and the other in which you are active. The passive aspect is usually referred to as the 'tablework', while the active aspect is called 'mentastics'.

Each session usually lasts 60 to 90 minutes. During the passive part of the session, for which you can either wear loose comfortable clothing or undress down to your underwear, you will be asked to lie on a comfortably padded table. The practitioner will then assess you and move you in ways that you naturally move, using gentle movements such as rocking and stretching, and in such a way that you will experience the feeling of moving effortlessly. While giving this part of the treatment, the practitioner maintains a soft focus of awareness of you and what is happening in your body. Instead of increasing pressure in an area of tension, the practitioner lightens his or her touch, with the aim of transmitting a sense of freedom to you. This quality of effortless movement is maintained and reinforced by mentastics, which are simple movements and awareness taught in the session that you can do on your own. The idea is to practise the movements during your daily activities, so that they become part of your life.

Practitioners claim that, by using gentle, non-intrusive, natural movements, Tragerwork helps to release deep-seated physical and mental patterns that may have developed in response to accidents, illnesses, or any kind of physical or emotional trauma, including the stress of everyday life. They also claim that it facilitates deep relaxation, increased physical mobility and mental clarity. One study found that Tragerwork can ease pain, while another found that it eased symptoms of lung disease after only two weeks of therapy.

The movements are never forced so should not cause pain or discomfort. There are no known safety concerns with Tragerwork.

Finding a practitioner

Certified practitioners of Tragerwork must have successfully completed the certification programme of the Trager International*, and have maintained continuing education, and met the other requirements of the Institute. The Trager Institute has a database of all Certified Practitioners worldwide, of which there are now over 800. If you have any question about someone's credentials, you are advised to contact the Institute for verification. The Trager International Practitioner certification programmes consist of a combination of hands-on training, fieldwork, and supervised tutorials which take from about 500 to 1,000 hours. All British practitioners are registered with Trager UK★. Contact an individual practitioner to find out how much a session costs.

Visualisation

Also known as imagery or guided imagery, visualisation is the controlled use of positive mental images and thoughts for therapeutic purposes. The aim is to reduce any negative emotions and fears you might have and to enhance your self-image. Some people also use visualisation to help create what they want in life. Visualisation has been shown to affect the physiology of the body, so making it a useful mind-body bridge. It is used to promote the body's natural healing processes and also to provide insight and improve self-awareness.

Visualisation works first by using positive and calming images and thoughts, which are chosen for their potential to alter mood, and second by directing thoughts away from any current problems or illnesses and towards a desired outcome. The theory is that whatever we visualise or think about, we are more likely to create in our bodies and in our lives. A visualisation can be self-directed, for example, if you want to be more relaxed, imagining a calm and peaceful environment, such as a beautiful lake, forest glade or sunny meadow, can slow your breathing down and help you feel calmer. A visualisation can also be guided by a therapist or followed from a tape or CD. You can practise visualisation on your own or within a group. Sessions tend to last between 30 and 60 minutes.

It is not known scientifically exactly how visualisation works, but it is thought to encourage activity in the higher centres of the right side of the brain, which relates to creativity and emotions. In turn, this sends messages to the hormonal system and autonomic nervous system of the body, which controls unconscious physiological functions such as how fast the heart beats and sweating.

Therapeutically, visualisation is used to treat psychological symptoms such as anxiety and depression, stress-related physical symptoms, pain and cancer. Cancer patients, for example, are asked to imagine their own version of immune system cells attacking their cancer cells, and to see their immune cells and the cancer treatments that they are having as strong and powerful, while imagining the cancer cells as weak. The visualisation culminates with the destruction of the cancer cells and the healing of the body. There is no scientific evidence that this visualisation improves the outcome of people with cancer, but patients have reported that it helps relieve anxiety and pain, improves their toleration of the cancer therapy, and also helps them to cope better with their illness. There have been some preliminary studies suggesting that visualisation may increase a person's immune response, but the results need confirming. There are no known safety concerns, but people with psychoses or personality disorders should be supervised.

Finding a practitioner

Visualisation is used by psychotherapists and counsellors, and may also be used by some complementary therapists, healers and conventional healthcare practitioners. It also forms a part of many relaxation therapies.

Glossary

Adrenaline (epinephrine) a hormone (*q.v.*) produced in the body by the adrenal glands in response to exercise, stress or emotions such as fear.

Antioxidant a substance that finds and mops up free radicals in the body. Free radicals are molecules that our bodies make as part of the defence against bacteria. Levels of free radicals can rise owing to cigarette smoke, chemicals and industrial pollution. Although free radicals 'live' only for a few seconds, they can damage DNA (genetic material) in cells and affect cholesterol so that it is more likely to stick to artery walls. These actions can make us more susceptible to cancer and to heart and circulatory disorders. Vitamins A, C and E are examples of antioxidants.

Aura an energy field said to be emitted by all living things. Some healers claim to be able to see auras, and to assess people's health from them.

Autoimmune disease a disease in which the body produces antibodies that attack its own tissues, for example, rheumatoid arthritis.

Autonomic nervous system the part of the body's nervous system that works automatically to regulate the heart and circulation, breathing, digestion, waste excretion and glands. It has two parts: the parasympathetic (q.v.) and sympathetic (q.v.) nervous systems.

Biopsychosocial an approach used in orthodox medicine that takes into account the psychological and sociocultural needs of a person, in addition to his or her biological needs.

Enzymes substances made by cells in the body that act as catalysts to make certain biological processes take place.

Hormones substances produced by glands (e.g. the thyroid) in the body that are vital for the normal functioning and growth of the body.

Immune system the body's defence system against invading microbes such as bacteria and viruses, and other foreign substances.

Lymphatic system the system in the body responsible for carrying and filtering lymph, a colourless fluid similar to blood plasma. Lymph contains white blood cells and bathes all the tissues of the body.

Neurotransmitters chemicals produced in the body at nerve endings, which transmit nerve signals from one nerve to another or to muscles.

Parasympathetic nervous system the part of the autonomic nervous system (*q.v.*) that inhibits activity in the body, in opposition to the sympathetic nervous system (*q.v.*). Most daily bodily functions, such as excretion and digestion, are controlled by this system.

Psychoneuroimmunology (PNI) an area of orthodox medical research that investigates the links between the mind (psycho), the brain and nervous system (neuro), and the body's natural defences (immuno), and which claims that the mind and body communicate with each other via a two-way flow of hormones (*q.v.*) and neurotransmitters (*q.v.*).

Sympathetic nervous system the part of the autonomic nervous system (*q.v.*) that stimulates a particular organ in the body to work harder, as opposed to the parasympathetic nervous system (*q.v.*), which inhibits activity. It controls bodily functions during exercise or when one is experiencing an emotion such as anger or fright, for example, making the heart beat harder and faster.

Addresses

General

Action for Victims of Medical Accidents
Bank Chambers
1 London Road
Forest Hill
London SE23 3TP
Tel: 020-8291 2793

British Complementary Medicine Association
PO Box 2074
Seaford BN25 1HQ
Tel: (0845) 345 5977
Website: www.bcma.co.uk

British Holistic Medical Association
59 Lansdowne Place
Hove
East Sussex BN3 1FL
Tel: (01273) 725951
Website: www.bhma.org

British Medical Association
BMA House
Tavistock Square
London WC1H 9JP
Tel: 020-7387 4499
Website: www.bma.org.uk

Clinical Negligence Panel
Ipsley Court
Redditch B98 0TD
Tel: (01527) 504433

Community Legal Service
Selborne House
54–60 Victoria Street
London SW1A 6QW
Directory line: (0845) 608 1122
Website: www.justask.org.uk

Council for Complementary and Alternative Medicine
63 Jeddo Road
London W12 6HQ
Tel: 020-8735 0632

Foundation for Integrated Medicine
12 Chillingworth Road
London N7 8QJ
Tel: 020-7619 6140
Website: www.fimed.org

General Medical Council
178 Great Portland Street
London W1W 5JE
Tel: 020-7580 7642
Website: www.gmc-uk.org

Health Service Ombudsman
Website: www.ombudsman.org.uk

Institute for Complementary Medicine
PO Box 194
London SE16 1QZ
Tel: 020-7237 5165
Website: www.icmedicine.co.uk

Law Society
Accident Line: (0500) 192939

Legal Services Commission
85 Gray's Inn Road
London WC1X 8TX
Tel: 020-7759 0000
Leafletline: (0845) 300 0343
Website: www.legalservices.gov.uk

Medical Research Council
20 Park Crescent
London W1B 1AL
Tel: 020-7636 5422
Website: www.mrc.ac.uk

Medicines Control Agency
1 Nine Elms Lane
London SW8 5NQ
Tel: 020-7273 0000
Website: www.mca.gov.co.uk

*The National Center for
Complementary and Alternative
Medicine*
Website: www.nccam.nih.gov

Natural Medicines Society
PO Box 134
Chessington
Surrey KT9 1HP
Tel: (0870) 240 4784
Website: www.the-nms.org.uk

*Research Council for Complementary
Medicine*
60 Great Ormond Street
London WC1N 3JF
Tel: 020-7833 8897
Website: www.rccm.org.uk

Main therapies

Acupuncture

British Acupuncture Council
63 Jeddo Road
London W12 9HQ
Tel: 020-8735 0400
Website: www.acupuncture.org.uk

British Medical Acupuncture Society
12 Marbury House
Higher Whitley
Warrington WA4 4AW
Tel: (01925) 730727
Website:
www.medical-acupuncture.co.uk

*The Acupuncture Association of
Chartered Physiotherapists*
Portcullis
Castle Street
Mere
Wiltshire BA12 6JE
Tel: (01747) 861151
Website: www.aacp.uk.com

Alexander technique

*Society of Teachers of the Alexander
Technique*
129 Camden Mews
London NW1 9AH
Tel: 020-7482 5159
Website: www.stat.org.uk

Aromatherapy

Aromatherapy Organisations Council
PO Box 19834
London SE25 6WF
Tel: 020-8251 7912
Website: www.aocuk.net

Aromatherapy Trade Council
PO Box 387
Ipswich
Suffolk IP2 9AN
Send an sae for a general information booklet

Autogenic therapy

British Autogenic Society
Royal London Homeopathic
Hospital
Great Ormond Street
London WC1N 3HR
Website: www.autogenic-
therapy.org.uk

Biofeedback

Biofeedback Foundation of Europe
PO Box 75416
1070 AK Amsterdam
The Netherlands
(00 31) 20 44 22 631
Website: www.bfe.org

Chiropractic

General Chiropractic Council
344–354 Gray's Inn road
London WC1X 8BP
Tel: 020-7713 5155
Website: www.gcc-uk.org

McTimoney Chiropractic Association
21 High Street
Eynsham OX8 1HE
Tel: (01865) 880974

National Back Pain Association
16 Elmtree Road
Teddington TW11 8ST
Tel: 020-8977 5474
Website: www.backpain.org

Healing

British Alliance of Healing Associations
Website: www.bahahealing.co.uk

Confederation of Healing Organisations
27 Montefiore Court
Stamford Hill
London N16 5TY
Tel: 020-8800 3569

Doctor-Healer Network
See Confederation of Healing Organisations

National Federation of Spiritual Healers
Old Manor Farm Studio
Church Street
Sunbury-on-Thames
Surrey TW16 6RG
Tel: (0845) 123 2777
Website: www.nfsh.org.uk

Reiki Association
Cornbrook Bridge House
Cornbrook
Clee Hill
Ludlow SY8 3QQ
Tel: (01584) 891197

Herbalism

Ayurvedic Medical Association UK
59 Dulverton Road
South Croydon
Surrey CR2 8PJ
Tel: 020-8682 3876
Email: dr_nsmoorthy@hotmail.com

British Ayurvedic Medical Council
47 Nottingham Place
London W1M 3FE
Tel: 020-7224 6070

European Herbal Practitioners Association
45A Corsica Street
London N5 1JT
Tel: 020-7354 5067
Website:
www.users.globalnet.co.uk/~ehpa

National Institute of Medical Herbalists
56 Longbrook Street
Exeter EX4 6AH
Tel: (01392) 426022
Website: www.nimh.org.uk

Register of Chinese Herbal Medicine
Office 5, Ferndale Business Centre
1 Exeter Street
Norwich NR2 4QB
Tel: (01603) 623994
Website: www.rchm.co.uk

Homeopathy

Faculty of Homeopathy and British Homeopathic Association
15 Clerkenwell Close
London EC1R 0AA
Tel: 020-7566 7800
Website: www.trusthomeopathy.org

Society of Homeopaths
4a Artizan Road
Northampton NN1 4HU
Tel: (01604) 621400
Website: www.homeopathy-soh.org

Hypnotherapy

British Society of Experimental and Clinical Hypnosis
Dept of Clinical Oncology
Derbyshire Royal Infirmary
London Road
Derby DE1 2QY

British Society of Medical and Dental Hypnosis
4 Kirkwood Avenue
Cookridge
Leeds LS16 7JU
Tel: (07000) 560309
Website: www.bsmdh.org

Central Register of Advanced Hypnotherapists
PO Box 14526
London N4 2WG
Tel: 020-7354 9938
Website:
www.n-shap-ericksonian.co.uk

National Register of Hypnotherapists and Psychotherapists
Room B
12 Cross Street
Nelson
Lancashire BB9 7EN
Tel: (01282) 716839
Website: www.nrhp.co.uk

Massage therapy

British Massage Therapy Council
17 Rymers Lane
Oxford OX4 3JU
Tel: (01865) 774123
Website: www.bmtc.co.uk

London School of Sports Massage
28 Station Parade
Willesden Green
London NW2 4NX
Tel: 020-8452 8855

Massage Therapy Institute of Great Britain
PO Box 2726
London NW2 4NR
Tel: 020-7724 4105

Register of Tuina and Thai Massage Practitioners
Bodyharmonics Centre
54 Flecker's Drive
Hatherley
Cheltenham GL51 5DB
Tel: (01242) 582168

Shiatsu Society
Eastlands Court
St Peter's Road
Rugby
Warwick CV21 3QP
Tel: (01788) 555051
Website: www.shiatsu.org

Sports Massage Association
40 Nottingham Place
London W1U 5NX
Tel: 020-7908 3639

Naturopathy

General Council and Register of Naturopaths
British Naturopathic Association
Goswell House
2 Goswell Road
Street BA16 0JG
Tel: (01458) 840072
Website: www.naturopathy.org.uk

Nutritional therapy

British Association of Nutritional Therapists
Monomark House
27 Old Gloucester Street
London WC1N 3XX
Tel: (0870) 606 1284

British Dietetic Association
5th floor, Charles House
148/9 Great Charles Street
Queensway
Birmingham B3 3HT
Tel: 0121-200 8080
Website: www.bda.uk.com

British Society for Allergy, Environmental and Nutritional Medicine
PO Box 7
Knighton
Powys LD7 1WP
Tel: (01547) 550380
Website: www.jnem.demon.co.uk

Osteopathy

Craniosacral Therapy Association of the UK
Monomark House
27 Old Gloucester Street
London WC1N 3XX
Tel: (07000) 784735
Website: www.craniosacral.co.uk

General Osteopathic Council
Osteopathy House
176 Tower Bridge Road
London SE1 3LU
Tel: 020-7357 6655
Website: www.osteopathy.org.uk

National Back Pain Association
(see Chiropractic)

Reflexology

Association of Reflexologists
Monomark House
27 Old Gloucester Street
London WC1N 3XX
Tel: (0870) 567 3320
Website: www.reflexology.org/aor

British Reflexology Association
Monks Orchard
Whitbourne
Worcester WR6 5RB
Tel: (01886) 821207
Website: www.britreflex.co.uk

International Federation of Reflexologists
76–78 Edridge Road
Croydon
Surrey CR0 1EF
Tel: 020-8645 9134
Website: www.reflexology-ifr.com

Reflexology Forum
PO Box 2367
South Croydon
Surrey CR2 7ZE
Tel: (0800) 037 0130
Email: reflexologyforum@aol.com

Reflexologists' Society
135 Collins Meadow
Harlow
Essex CM19 4EJ
Tel: (01279) 421682

Relaxation therapy and meditation techniques

Friends of the Western Buddhist Order
London Buddhist Centre
51 Roman Road
London E2 0HU
Tel: 020-8981 1225

School of Meditation
158 Holland Park Avenue
London W11 4UH
Tel: 020-7603 6116

Transcendental Meditation
Freepost
London SW1P 4YY
Tel: (08705) 143733
Website: www.transcendental-meditation.org.uk

Yoga

British Wheel of Yoga
1 Hamilton Place
Boston Road
Sleaford NG34 7ES
Tel: (01529) 306851
Website: www.bwy.org.uk

Iyengar Yoga Institute
223a Randolph Avenue
London W9 1NL
Tel: 020-7624 3080
Website: www.iyi.org.uk

Sivananda Yoga Vedanta Centre
51 Felsham Road
London SW15 1AX
Tel: 020-8780 0160
Website: www.sivananda.org

Yoga Biomedical Trust/Yoga Therapy Centre
90–92 Pentonville Road
Islington
London N1 9HS
Tel: 020-7419 7911 *(Thurs & Fri)*
Website: www.yogatherapy.org

Diagnostic alternatives

Dowsing and radionics

British Society of Dowsers
Sycamore Barn
Hastingleigh
Ashford
Kent TN25 5HW
Tel: (01233) 750253
Website: www.britishdowsers.org

Radionics Association
Baerlein House
Goose Green
Deddington
Oxford OX5 0SZ
Tel: (01869) 338852
Website: www.radionic.co.uk

Iridology

Guild of Naturopathic Iridologists
94 Grosvenor Road
London SW1V 3LF
Tel: 020-7821 0255
Website: www.gni-international.org

International Association of Clinical Iridologists
853–5 Finchley Road
London NW1 8LX

Kinesiology

Association of Systematic Kinesiology
39 Browns Road
Surbiton KT5 8ST
Tel: 020-8399 3215
Website: www.kinesiology.co.uk

Kinesiology Federation
PO Box 17153
Edinburgh EH11 3WQ
Tel: (08700) 113545

Kirlian photography

Kirlian Research Ltd
25–27 Oxford Street
London W1R 1RR
Tel: 020-7287 7980
Website: www.kirlian.co.uk

Other therapies

Anthroposophical medicine

Anthroposophical Medical Association
Park Attwood Clinic
Trimpley
Bewdley DY12 1RE
Tel: (01299) 861444

Art therapy

British Association of Art Therapists
Mary Ward House
5 Tavistock Place
London W1H 9SN
020-7383 3774

Bowen technique

Bowen Association UK
PO Box 4358
Dorchester
Dorset DT1 3BA
Tel: (0700) 269 8324
Website: www.bowen-technique.co.uk

Bowen Therapists European Register
38 Portway
Frome
Somerset BA11 1QU
Website:
www.thebownetechnique.com

Chelation therapy

Arterial Health Foundation
PO Box 8
Atherton
Manchester M46 9FY
Tel: (01942) 878400

Colonic irrigation

Association and Register of Colon Hydrotherapists
16 Drummond Ride
Tring
Herts HP23 5DE
Tel: (01442) 827687
Website:
www.colonic-association.com

Colour therapy

International Association of Colour Therapy
46 Cottenham Road
Histon
Cambridge CB4 9ES
Website: www.
internationalassociationofcolour.com

Crystal healing

Affiliation of Crystal Healing Organisations
PO Box 100
Exminster
Exeter EX6 8YT
Tel: (01479) 841450
Website: www.crystal-healing.org

Dance and drama therapy

Association for Dance Movement Therapy
c/o Quaker Meeting House
Wedmore Vale
Bristol BS3 5HX
Website: www.dmtuk.demon.co.uk

British Association of Drama Therapists
4 Sunnydale Villas
Durlston Road
Swanage BN19 2HY

Feldenkrais method

Feldenkrais Guild UK
c/o The Bothy
Auchlunies Walled Garden
Aberdeen AB12 5YS
Tel: (07000) 785506
Website: www.feldenkrais.co.uk

Flotation therapy

Floatation Tank Association
7A Clapham Common Southside
London SW4 7AA
Tel: 020-7627 4962
Website:
www.floatationtankassociation.net

Flower remedies

British Flower and Vibrational Essences Association
PO Box 33
Exmouth
Devon EX8 1YY
Tel: (07986) 512064
Website: www.bfvea.com

Dr Edward Bach Centre
Mount Vernon
Sotwell
Wallingford OX10 0PZ
Tel: (01491) 834678
Website: www.bachcentre.com

Hellerwork

European Hellerwork Association
Thornfield
Stretton on Fosse
Moreton in Marsh
Gloucestershire GL56 9RA
Tel: (01608) 662828
Website: www.hellerwork-europe.com

Hellerwork International
Website: www.hellerwork.com

Holotropic breathwork and rebirthing

Association for Holotropic Breathwork International
Website: www.breathwork.com

British Rebirth Society
6 Belsize Park Gardens
London NW3 4LD
Tel: (0845) 458 1050

Transpersonal Training and Holotropic Breathwork
Website: www.holotropic.com

Light therapy

SAD Association
PO Box 989
Steyning BN44 3HG
Website: www.sada.org.uk

Magnetic therapy

British Biomagnetic Association
31 St Marychurch Road
Torquay TQ1 3JF
Tel: (01803) 293346

Metamorphic technique

Metamorphic Association
67 Ritherdon Road
London SW17 8QE
Tel: 020-8672 5951

Music therapy

Association of Professional Music Therapists
26 Hamlyn Road
Glastonbury
Somerset BA6 8HT
Tel: (01458) 834919
Website: www.apmt.org.uk

British Society for Music Therapy
25 Rosslyn Avenue
East Barnet EN4 8DH
Tel: 020-8368 8879
Website: www.bsmt.org.uk

Polarity therapy

Federation of Polarity Training
7 Nunney Close
Golden Valley
Cheltenham GL51 0TU
Tel: (01242) 52352

UK Polarity Therapy Association
Monomark House
27 Old Gloucester St
London WC1N 3XX
Tel: (0700) 705 2748
Website: www.ukpta.org.uk

Rolfing

Rolf Institute
PO Box 14793
London SW1V 2WB
Tel: 0117-946 6374
Website: www.rolf.org

European Rolfing Association
Website: www.rolfing.org

Sound therapy

The Listening Centre
The Maltings Studio
16A Station Street
Lewes
East Sussex BN7 2DB
Tel: (01273) 474877

T'ai chi and Qigong

T'ai Chi Union
1 Littlemill Drive
Crookston
Glasgow G53 7GE
Tel: 0141-810 3482
Website: www.taichiunion.com

UK T'ai Chi Association
PO Box 159
Bromley BR1 3XX
Tel: 020-8289 5166
Website: www.taichi-europe.com

Qigong Centre
PO Box 59
Altrincham WA15 8ES
Tel: 0161-929 4485
Website: www.qimagazine.com

Tragerwork

Trager International
Website: www.trager.com

Trager UK
13 Sycamore Close
Tilbury RM18 7TB
Tel: (01273) 411193
Website: www.trager.co.uk

Index

Page references in **bold** type indicate the main entry for a therapy

WHICH? BOOKS

The following titles were available as this book went to press.

General (legal, financial, practical etc)

Be Your Own Financial Adviser	448 pages	£10.99
420 Legal Problems Solved	352 pages	£9.99
Rip Off Britain – and how to beat it	256 pages	£5.99
What to Do When Someone Dies	192 pages	£9.99
The Which? Computer Troubleshooter	192 pages	£12.99
Which? Way to Buy, Own and Sell a Flat	352 pages	£10.99
Which? Way to Buy, Sell and Move House	320 pages	£10.99
Which? Way to Clean It	256 pages	£9.99
Which? Way to Drive Your Small Business	240 pages	£10.99
Which? Way to Manage Your Time – and Your Life	208 pages	£9.99
Which? Way to Save and Invest	352 pages	£14.99
Which? Way to Save Tax	320 pages	£14.99
Wills and Probate	192 pages	£10.99
Make Your Own Will Action Pack	28 pages	£10.99

A5 wallet with forms and 28-page book inside

The Which? Guide to:

Baby Products	240 pages	£9.99
Changing Careers	352 pages	£10.99
Choosing a Career	336 pages	£9.99
Choosing a School	336 pages	£10.99
Computers	352 pages	£10.99
Computers for Small Businesses	352 pages	£10.99
Divorce	368 pages	£10.99
Doing Your Own Conveyancing	208 pages	£9.99
Domestic Help	208 pages	£9.99
Employment	336 pages	£11.99
Gambling	288 pages	£9.99
Getting Married	256 pages	£9.99
Giving and Inheriting	256 pages	£9.99
Going Digital	272 pages	£10.99
Home Safety and Security	198 pages	£9.99
Insurance	320 pages	£10.99
Living Together	192 pages	£9.99
Money	448 pages	£9.99
Money on the Internet	256 pages	£9.99
Planning Your Pension	368 pages	£10.99
Renting and Letting	352 pages	£11.99
Shares	288 pages	£9.99
Shopping on the Internet	272 pages	£10.99
Starting Your Own Business	288 pages	£10.99
Working from Home	256 pages	£9.99

Health
The Which? Guide to:

Children's Health	288 pages	£9.99
Managing Back Trouble	160 pages	£9.99
Managing Stress	252 pages	£9.99
Men's Health	336 pages	£9.99
Personal Health	320 pages	£10.99
Women's Health	448 pages	£9.99
Which? Medicine	544 pages	£12.99

Gardening
The Gardening Which? Guide to:

Growing Your Own Vegetables (hardback)	224 pages	£18.99
(paperback)	224 pages	£12.99
Patio and Container Plants	224 pages	£17.99
Small Gardens	224 pages	£12.99
Successful Perennials	224 pages	£17.99
Successful Propagation	160 pages	£12.99
Successful Pruning	240 pages	£12.99
Successful Shrubs	224 pages	£12.99

Do-it-yourself

The Which? Book of Do-It-Yourself	320 pages	£14.99
The Which? Book of Plumbing and Central Heating	160 pages	£13.99
The Which? Book of Wiring and Lighting	160 pages	£16.99
Which? Way to Fix It	208 pages	£12.99

Travel/leisure

The Good Bed and Breakfast Guide	624 pages	£14.99
The Good Food Guide	768 pages	£15.99
The Good Skiing and Snowboarding Guide	384 pages	£15.99
The Good Walks Guide	320 pages	£13.99
The Which? Guide to Country Pubs	576 pages	£13.99
The Which? Guide to Pub Walks	256 pages	£9.99
The Which? Guide to Scotland	528 pages	£12.99
The Which? Guide to Tourist Attractions	544 pages	£12.99
The Which? Guide to Weekend Breaks in Britain	528 pages	£13.99
The Which? Hotel Guide	736 pages	£15.99
The Which? Wine Guide	512 pages	£14.99
Which? Holiday Destination	624 pages	£12.99

Available from bookshops, and by post from:
Which?, Dept BKLIST, Castlemead, Gascoyne Way, Hertford X, SG14 1LH
or phone FREE on (0800) 252100
quoting Dept BKLIST and your credit-card details